Contents

Preface   vii

About this book   viii

Q1   Define (a) standard deviation, (b) standard error of the   1
     mean and (c) 95% confidence interval

Q2   Define sensitivity, specificity and positive predictive   2
     value of screening

Q3   Write short notes on the factors determining drug penetration   3
     into the eye

Q4   Write short notes on drug metabolism   5

Q5   Describe the pupillary responses and their modification   7
     by drugs

Q6   List, with examples, pharmacological ways of lowering   9
     intraocular pressure

Q7   Write short notes on the pharmacology of cycloplegic drugs   11

Q8   Write short notes on carbonic anhydrase inhibitors   12

Q9   Write short notes on the side effects of β-blockers   14

Q10 Write short notes on the mode of action of drugs that   15
     lower blood glucose

Q11 Write short notes on the mode of action of drugs that lower   17
     blood pressure

Q12 Write short notes on the side effects of aminoglycosides   18

Q13 What are the side effects of corticosteroids?   19

Q14 What are the current therapeutic strategies in the human   21
     immunodeficiency virus (HIV)?

Q15 Write short notes comparing rods and cones   23

Q16 Describe the mechanisms regulating aqueous outflow   25

Q17 Describe the structures and relationships of different retinal   26
     ganglion cell types, including their connection to higher
     visual pathways

Q18 Write short notes on autoregulation of blood flow   28

Q19 Outline the differences between the sympathetic and   29
     parasympathetic branches of the autonomic nervous system

Q20 Write short notes on steroid receptors. Illustrate your answer   30
     with reference to the glucocorticoid receptor

Q21   Describe the physiological and pharmacological mechanisms   31
      involved in water transfer through tissue
Q22   Write short notes on endocytosis. Illustrate your answer with   33
      an example from the eye
Q23   Discuss mechanisms by which bacteria destroy tissue   34
Q24   List the ophthalmic manifestations of the acquired   35
      immunodeficiency syndrome (AIDS)
Q25   List the clinical manifestations of giant cell arteritis   37
Q26   Discuss the pathological effects of ionising radiation   38
Q27   Draw a diagram of the normal retinal capillary. How is the   39
      structure altered in diabetes?
Q28   Write short notes on the pathogenesis of atheromatous   40
      plaques
Q29   Describe the causes and effects of ulcers   42
Q30   What are free radicals? Write short notes explaining why   44
      retinal photoreceptors are particularly vulnerable to
      free radicals
Q31   Describe ways in which cells die   45
Q32   Write short notes on viral replication   46
Q33   Contrast Gram-negative and Gram-positive bacteria   47
Q34   Describe the chief mechanisms by which bacteria acquire   48
      resistance to antibiotics
Q35   Discuss the microbiology of *Pseudomonas aeruginosa*   49
Q36   What precautions would be taken to prevent spread of   50
      methicillin-resistant *Staphylococcus aureus* (MRSA) infection
      from patient to patient on an ophthalmic ward?
Q37   Write short notes on the principles of sterilisation   52
Q38   Compare and contrast bacteria, viruses and chlamydia   53
Q39   Write short notes on genetic linkage analysis. Give an   54
      example
Q40   Discuss the genetic mechanisms involved in neoplasia   55
Q41   Write short notes on prenatal testing   57
Q42   Write short notes on the polymerase chain reaction   58
Q43   What is a chromosomal translocation? Illustrate your answer   59
      with an example associated with ocular disease
Q44   Describe the causes and effects of occlusive disease occurring   60
      in muscular arteries and arterioles
Q45   List the major roles of complement   62
Q46   Describe the structure and function of immunoglobulins   63
Q47   Write short notes on histocompatibility antigens and list   65
      three examples of disease associations
Q48   Write short notes on the mechanism of allograft rejection   67

Short Answer Questions for the MRCOphth Part 1

Nathaniel Knox Cartwright
Senior House Officer
Bristol Eye Hospital
Bristol, UK

and

Petros Carvounis
Chief Resident
Department of Ophthalmology
The George Washington University
Washington DC, USA

Radcliffe Publishing
Oxford ● Seattle

Radcliffe Publishing Ltd
18 Marcham Road
Abingdon
Oxon OX14 1AA
United Kingdom

www.radcliffe-oxford.com
Electronic catalogue and worldwide online ordering facility.

British Library Cataloguing in Publication Data

A catalogue record for this book is available from the British Library.

ISBN 1 85775 884 6

Typeset by Aarontype Ltd, Easton, Bristol
Printed and bound by TJ International Ltd, Padstow, Cornwall

Q49 Describe how antigen is presented to T lymphocytes 68

Q50 Discuss the local and systemic effects of neoplasia 69

Q51 Compare and contrast the innate and adaptive immune 70
responses

Q52 Describe the histology of hypertensive vasculopathy 72

Q53 Describe the structure and function of mitochondria 73

Q54 Write short notes on the bony anatomy of the orbit 74

Q55 Write short notes on the blood supply to the anterior 76
segment of the eye

Q56 Outline the blood supply to the visual pathway 78

Q57 List the actions of the extraocular muscles and list the 79
differences between extraocular muscles and other skeletal
muscles

Q58 Write short notes on the crystallins 80

Q59 Write short notes on carbohydrate metabolism in the lens 81

Q60 List, with a brief explanation, the protective mechanisms 82
against oxidative damage to the lens

Q61 Draw a dark adaptation curve and identify the component 83
parts and their significance

Q62 Describe the mechanisms of visual adaptation 85

Q63 What is known of the function of retinal pigment 87
epithelial cells?

Q64 Write short notes on the electrophysiological investigations 88
of the visual pathway

Q65 Describe the absorption of ultraviolet, visible and infrared 91
light by the eye and discuss their harmful effects

Q66 Describe the retinotopic organisation of the visual pathway. 93
Use an image in the left superior visual field as an example

Q67 Write short notes on the classification of visual acuity 95

Q68 Discuss the cortical contribution to visual function 96

Q69 Write short notes on the normal visual field and how it can 98
be measured

Q70 Write short notes on the principles of intraocular pressure 100
measurement

Q71 Discuss the mechanisms of aqueous secretion and their 101
modification by drugs

Q72 Write short notes on the supranuclear control of eye 103
movements

Q73 Describe the mechanism of colour perception 105

Q74 Draw a cross-section of the upper eyelid. Label all important 107
structures and write short notes on each

Q75 Describe the structure and function of the conjunctiva 109

Q76   Draw a diagram of the anterior chamber drainage angle and   110
      write short notes on the anatomy of the structure
Q77   Describe the structure and function of the ciliary body   112
Q78   Describe the lacrimal gland. Include a short note on its   114
      development
Q79   Discuss the anatomy of the cerebellum, including its blood   115
      supply and neuronal connections
Q80   Write short notes on the anatomy of the third cranial nerve   117
      nucleus
Q81   Write short notes on the third cranial nerve   118
Q82   Write short notes on the fourth cranial nerve   120
Q83   Give an account of the origin, course, relations and functions   122
      of the sixth cranial nerve
Q84   Give an account of the structure and function of the primary   124
      visual cortex and its neuronal connections
Q85   Write short notes on the paranasal air sinuses   126
Q86   Write short notes on the ventricles of the brain   128
Q87   Write short notes on the major photochemical events   130
      involved in phototransduction
Q88   Write short notes on retinal neurotransmitters   132
Q89   List the factors that determine corneal hydration   134
Q90   Discuss the anatomical features of the extraocular muscles   135
Q91   What are the Golgi apparatus? How are they involved in the   137
      secretion of proteins? Describe this process in relation to
      mast cells
Q92   Compare and contrast the magnocellular and parvocellular   138
      pathways
Q93   Write short notes on the development of the cornea   140
Q94   Write short notes on the prenatal development of the lens.   141
      Use annotated diagrams where possible
Q95   Write short notes on the early development of the vitreous   143
Q96   Write short notes on the development of the retina   144

Index   145

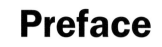

Preface

This book is based on the revision notes we made while studying for the short answer paper of the Part 1 MRCOphth examination. Our aim has been to produce 'exam style' model answers to many of the most frequently asked questions. We do not pretend that this is a comprehensive text or that buying it will substitute for investing many hours in revision. Despite that, we are proud of what we have produced and hope you will find it a useful revision aid. Good luck!

Nathaniel Knox Cartwright
November 2004

About this book

This book is targeted at those revising for the short answer paper of the Part 1 MRCOphth examination in the United Kingdom and similar examinations elsewhere. More than 90 model answers to typical basic science short answer questions are presented, mostly in note and table form, each with a level of detail appropriate to the format of the examination.

Short Answer Questions

Q1   Define (a) standard deviation, (b) standard error of the mean and (c) 95% confidence interval

(a)   **Standard deviation (SD)** is a **statistical measure of the spread** of a series of values. SD is the square root of variance. In a given population SD varies little with sample size. In a normally distributed population 66% of values lie within 1 SD of the mean and 95% within 1.96 SD. The smaller the SD the more closely grouped the values.

(b)   **Standard error of the mean (SEM)** is a measure of **how close the mean of a sample is to the true population mean**. It is equal to the standard deviation divided by the square root of the number of values $(SEM = SD/\sqrt{n})$. SEM falls as the sample size increases and is smaller in more closely grouped samples. If the SEM is small the calculated mean of the sample is likely to be close to the true population mean.

(c)   The **95% confidence interval (CI)** is the **range of values** within which it can be said that 95% of the time the **true value of a measurement**, for example the population mean, lies. As described above, in normally distributed populations confidence intervals are based on the SD.

Q2   Define sensitivity, specificity and positive predictive value of screening

A screening test is meant to establish whether a person has a particular condition or not. Ideally, such a test would be positive for all people who actually have the condition and negative for all those without it. In reality, some people with the condition test negative for it ('false negatives') and some people who do not have the condition test positive for it ('false positives').

Sensitivity, specificity and positive and negative predictive value are all statistical measures which help interpret the significance of a particular test result.

Sensitivity is a measure of a test's ability to identify true disease. Sensitivity is expressed as a percentage and calculated by dividing the number of true positive results by the total number of people with the disease (true positives + false negatives). Tests with high sensitivity have low false negative rates.

Specificity is a measure of a test's ability to correctly identify those without disease. Like sensitivity, it is independent of disease prevalence and is expressed as a percentage. Specificity is calculated by dividing the number of true negatives by the total number of people without the disease (true negatives + false positives).

Positive predictive value (PPV) is the measure of how likely someone with a positive test result is to actually have the disease. PPV equates to the number of true positives divided by the number who actually have the disease (true positives + false negatives). PPV varies with disease prevalence.

Q3   Write short notes on the factors determining drug penetration into the eye

Drug properties, mode of administration, natural ocular barriers and the presence of ocular inflammation all influence drug penetration into the eye.

Drug properties

- Smaller molecules penetrate better than larger molecules. Most antibiotics are large molecules.
- Lipid-soluble drugs penetrate into the eye better than water-soluble drugs.
- Highly protein-bound drugs do not penetrate well.

Mode of administration

- In most cases topical formulations allow adequate intraocular concentrations of drugs to be reached whilst avoiding excessive systemic absorption and concomitant side effects.
- Blink rate, conjunctival sac volume, conjunctival: corneal area ratio and the rate of tear production all influence absorption of topically applied drugs.
- Absorption is increased when preparations are used which prolong the time the drug spends in the conjunctival sac. Most simply this can be achieved by making the preparation more viscous but other methods, such as drug-impregnated soft contact lenses, also exist.
- Direct administration of a drug to the intended site of action by injection bypasses natural ocular barriers and allows very high local drug levels to be achieved.
- Drugs may be administered to the eye by subconjunctival, sub-Tenon's, peribulbar, retrobulbar and intravitreal injection.

Natural ocular barriers

- Epithelial barrier of the cornea:
  - major barrier to entry of most topically applied drugs
  - provides most resistance to lipophilic compounds but as the cornea is a 'fat–water–fat' sandwich, drugs which are able to exist in both ionised and non-ionised forms are best able to penetrate the cornea

  – barrier function can be disrupted by infection, by trauma and by certain drugs (e.g. local anaesthetics).
- Aqueous–vitreous barrier:
  – bulk flow of aqueous into the anterior chamber and the presence of an intact lens and zonules retard diffusion of drugs from the anterior segment to the vitreous.
- Blood–retinal and blood–aqueous barriers:
  – limit entry of drugs into the eye from the systemic circulation
  – small lipophilic molecules penetrate best
  – when given systemically, higher peak drug levels lead to higher intraocular levels: bolus administration is preferable to continuous administration
  – may be broken down in inflammatory conditions such as uveitis.

Q4   Write short notes on drug metabolism

Overview

- Most drugs are metabolised in the liver, although drug metabolism does occur to a lesser extent in other organs:
  - suxamethonium in the plasma
  - vitamin D in the kidneys
  - neurotransmitters at synapses.
- Most locally administered ophthalmic medications are metabolised in the liver after removal from the eye in the bloodstream.
- The eye, in particular the ciliary body, has a limited capacity to break down certain drugs.

Phase I reactions

- Involve chemical alteration of a drug's basic structure commonly by oxidation, reduction or hydrolysis.
- Oxidation reactions are subdivided by whether they are effected by cytochrome-linked mixed function oxidases, the most important of which is cytochrome P450.
- Conversion of ethanol to acetaldehyde is a phase I reaction.

Phase 2 reactions

- Involve conjugation, for example by sulphation, glucuronidation, methylation or acetylation.
- Usually follow phase I reactions but some drugs can be conjugated directly.
- End products are generally pharmacologically inactive and water-soluble.
- Paracetamol is conjugated by glucuronidation.

Outcome

- Metabolism usually produces inactive compounds capable of being excreted by the kidneys.

- However, some drugs produce toxic metabolites:
  - lignocaine is metabolised to monoethylglycylxylidide and glycylxylidide
  - in overdose, paracetamol forms toxic metabolites when its normal metabolic pathways are saturated.
- Some drugs are given as pro-drugs which are themselves inactive but which produce active metabolites:
  - talampicillin is better absorbed than ampicillin, to which it is metabolised.

Variables

- Genetic: *AD*
  - N-acetyltransferase is an autosomally dominantly inherited hepatic enzyme that acetylates drugs, including isoniazid. 60% of Europeans are slow acetylators and require lower doses of such drugs and are more susceptible to their side effects.
- Drugs are metabolised more slowly at the extremes of age:
  - chloramphenicol is metabolised by UDP [uridine 5'-diphosphate] glucoronyl transferase. Neonates have low levels of this enzyme and weight-adjusted doses of chloramphenicol which would not be toxic to adults can lead to circulatory collapse and the 'grey baby syndrome'.
- Liver disease.
- Drug interactions, particularly for phase I reactions:
  - phenytoin, carbamazepine and rifampicin all induce cytochrome P450
  - chloramphenicol, warfarin and isoniazid all inhibit cytochrome P450.

Q5   Describe the pupillary responses and their modification by drugs

Overview

- Pupil diameter is under autonomic control:
  - the radially arranged dilator pupillae is sympathetically innervated
  - the circumferentially arranged sphincter pupillae muscle receives parasympathetic innervation and constricts the pupil.
- Normal pupillary responses are constriction to light and when looking at a near target.

Innervation

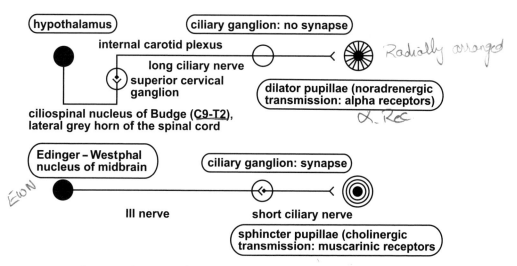

Figure 1   Schematic diagram of the innervation of sphincter and dilator pupillae muscles.

Pharmacological modification

Some drugs which affect pupillary reactions are listed below. Some act in more than one way.

Miotics (constrict the pupil)

- *Sympathetic antagonists*
    - central depressants − sedatives
    - blockers of superior cervical ganglion − hexamethonium, high-dose nicotine
    - prevention of noradrenaline release − guanethidine
    - prevention of noradrenaline storage − reserpine
    - α-receptor blockers − thymoxamine, phentolamine.
- *Parasympathetic agonists*
    - loss of supranuclear inhibition − opiates, barbiturates
    - stimulation of superior cervical ganglion − low-dose nicotine
    - acetylcholinesterase inhibitors − physostigmine, neostigmine, edrophonium
    - direct muscarinic stimulation − pilocarpine, carbachol
    - direct muscle fibre stimulation − histamine, prostaglandins.

Mydriatics (dilate the pupil)

- *Sympathetic agonists*
    - central stimulants − cocaine, caffeine, noradrenaline
    - stimulation of superior cervical ganglion − low-dose nicotine
    - stimulation of noradrenaline release − adrenaline, amphetamine, ephedrine
    - block of noradrenaline reuptake − cocaine
    - direct α-receptor stimulation − adrenaline, phenylephrine, ephedrine.
- *Parasympathetic antagonists*
    - supranuclear inhibition − cocaine, amphetamine
    - block ciliary ganglion − hexamethonium, high-dose nicotine
    - block acetylcholine release − botulinum toxin
    - block muscarinic cholinergic receptors − atropine, scopolamine, cyclopentolate, tropicamide, homatropine.

Q6   List, with examples, pharmacological ways of lowering intraocular pressure

Intraocular pressure (IOP) results from the balance between aqueous production and drainage within the relatively non-distensible globe. Aqueous is produced by the ciliary epithelium. The majority of aqueous drains via the trabecular meshwork into Schlemm's canal (conventional route); a proportion drains via the uveoscleral route (non-conventional route). Mean IOP is 16.5 mmHg with a standard deviation of 2.5 mmHg.

Many classes of drug reduce IOP:

- β-blockers (e.g. timolol):
  - reduce aqueous secretion by β_2-blockade
  - those with intrinsic sympathomimetic activity, such as carteolol, may have an additional neuroprotective effect in glaucoma by increasing optic nerve head blood flow
  - systemic side effects include bradycardia and bronchospasm
- α_2 -agonists (e.g. brimonidine):
  - reduce ciliary epithelium aqueous secretion
- muscarinic agonists (e.g. pilocarpine):
  - act on the ciliary spur to increase aqueous outflow by 'opening up' the trabecular meshwork
- prostaglandin F_2 $_\alpha$ analogues (e.g. latanoprost):
  - facilitate aqueous drainage via the non-conventional or uveoscleral route
  - can cause iris hyperpigmentation and eyelash growth
- carbonic anhydrase inhibitors (e.g. dorzolamide and acetazolamide):
  - act on the ciliary epithelium to reduce active secretion of aqueous
  - topical agents are a useful adjunct in the treatment of chronic open-angle glaucoma
  - systemic acetazolamide is administered in acute angle-closure glaucoma but its widespread side effects, including paraesthesias, hypokalaemia, nephrolithiasis and altered taste, usually prohibit long-term use
- α- and β-agonists (e.g. epinephrine):
  - facilitate outflow via the conventional route through an action on the trabecular meshwork
  - some reduce aqueous secretion
- osmotic agents (e.g. mannitol):
  - used to bring about rapid falls in IOP in acute angle-closure glaucoma
  - must be used with caution in those with renal or cardiac impairment
  - not suitable for long-term use

- **Na–K ATPase inhibitors**:
  - not available for clinical use
  - *in vitro* ouabain reduces active secretion of aqueous by the ciliary epithelium
- **systemic anti-hypertensive agents**:
  - drugs which reduce systemic blood pressure, and therefore episcleral venous pressure, increase aqueous drainage through the conventional route.

Q7 Write short notes on the pharmacology of cycloplegic drugs

Cycloplegic drugs prevent accommodation and focus on near objects by paralysing the ciliary muscle. All cycloplegic agents are anti-muscarinic drugs and also cause mydriasis. Not all mydriatics cause cycloplegia; sympatho-mimetic agents produce mydriasis but not cycloplegia.

The four most widely used cycloplegic agents are, in order of potency, atropine, cyclopentolate, tropicamide and homatropine. All are competitive inhibitors of acetylcholine at muscarinic receptors. They are affected by pigment binding: efficacy is reduced and latency of action increased in highly pigmented eyes. The mydriatic action of atropine is supplemented by direct stimulation of α-receptors on the dilator pupillae muscle.

Cycloplegic drugs are commonly used to dilate the pupil for fundus examination or photography, during cycloplegic refraction, to prevent synechiae formation in uveitis and to relieve the pain of ciliary muscle spasm.

Local side effects include irritation, hyperaemia, blurred vision, photophobia, raised intraocular pressure and precipitation of angle-closure glaucoma. Systemic side effects include fever, nausea, dry mouth, skin flushing, gastrointestinal upset, hypotension, urinary retention, arrhythmias, behavioural disturbances, ataxic dysarthria and seizures.

Table 1 gives the speed and duration of action of the four drugs mentioned above.

Table 1 Cycloplegic agents

	Max. mydriasis/min	Max. cycloplegia/min	Duration of action
Atropine	40	360	7–10 days
Homatropine	60	60	1–2 days
Cyclopentolate	60	60	12–24 hours
Tropicamide	40	30	3–4 hours

Q8 Write short notes on carbonic anhydrase inhibitors

Background

- Carbonic anhydrase is the enzyme which catalyses the reversible reaction $CO_2 + H_2O \leftrightarrow HCOO_3^- + H^+$.
- Type 2 carbonic anhydrase is present in the ciliary epithelium of the eye and is important in aqueous humour production.
- Inhibition of carbonic anhydrase reduces intraocular pressure.
- Carbonic anhydrase is also present in the renal tubules, red blood cells and gastric mucosa.
- Acetazolamide was the first oral carbonic anhydrase inhibitor (CAI) to be developed but it is very hydrophilic and does not penetrate the cornea well. For topical use, compounds such as dorzolamide have been developed.
- CAIs are sulphonamide derivatives: their use is contraindicated in those with sulphonamide hypersensitivity.

Systemic carbonic anhydrase inhibitors

- Oral carbonic anhydrase inhibitors can be used for short-term control of intraocular pressure but their wide range of side effects usually limits long-term use.
- Outside ophthalmology, CAIs are used to treat epilepsy and altitude sickness.
- Oral CAIs commonly cause circumoral and peripheral paraesthesias, anorexia, general malaise and altered taste.
- Additionally they may cause polyuria, hypokalaemia, urinary alkalisation, nephrolithiasis and metabolic acidosis.
- CAIs increase the risk of salicylate toxicity during concomitant aspirin therapy.
- Their most serious side effects include Stevens–Johnson syndrome, transaminitis and bone marrow suppression.
- CAIs are excreted in the urine and their dose should be reduced in renal failure.

Topical carbonic anhydrase inhibitors

- Topical agents are preferred for long-term ophthalmic use, having greater site specificity and a lower rate of systemic side effects.
- Commonly they cause headache, bitter taste (up to 25%), fatigue and paraesthesia.
- CAIs may cause local side effects such as burning, stinging, blepharoconjunctivitis and keratitis.

Q9   Write short notes on the side effects of β-blockers

Topical β-blockers are used to reduce intraocular pressure by reducing aqueous humour production by the ciliary epithelium. Systemic β-blockers are prescribed for a variety of mainly cardiovascular indications.

Systemic side effects

These can occur even with topical administration:

- fatigue
- hypotension, bradycardia and heart failure
  - concomitant calcium channel antagonist usage increases the risk of these side effects
- bronchospasm
  - particularly by non-cardioselective agents
- depression and nightmares
  - especially if lipid-soluble and able to cross the blood–brain barrier
- impotence and reduced libido.

Because β-blockers reduce glucose tolerance and mask the symptoms of hypoglycaemia they should be used with caution in diabetics.

Ocular side effects

These occur only with topical preparations:

- burning, stinging, erythema
- dry eyes
- allergic blepharoconjunctivitis
- occasional corneal disorders
- propranolol has membrane stabilising properties and causes corneal anaesthesia.

Q10   Write short notes on the mode of action of drugs that lower blood glucose

In all type 1 diabetics and some type 2 diabetics subcutaneous insulin injections are used to lower blood glucose. This insulin acts in the same ways as physiological insulin and there is a risk of hypoglycaemia.

Oral therapy is the mainstay of treatment of type 2 diabetes not controlled by diet alone. Drugs fall into two main groups: those which increase insulin release from the pancreas – secretagogues – and drugs which increase the action of insulin – biguanides.

Secretagogues

- First-line drugs for use in the non-obese type 2 diabetic.
- Act to increase insulin release by closing ATP-dependent K channels on β-islet cells in the pancreas.
- Side effects include weight gain and hypoglycaemia.
- Sulphonylureas are the main drugs in this group and they are excreted hepatically.
- Gliclazide is a short-acting sulphonylurea; longer-acting agents have fallen from favour due to their higher frequency of side effects.
- Recently, non-sulphonylurea secretagogues such as repaglinide have been developed. These act in the same way as sulphonylureas but their role has yet to be established.

Biguanides

- Metformin is the only biguanide in clinical use.
- Its exact mode of action is unknown but it increases the action of insulin, possibly by raising tissue insulin sensitivity.
- Metformin does not cause weight gain, probably due to the common side effects of nausea and vomiting, and so is the first-choice agent in the obese.
- It is renally excreted and may cause metabolic acidosis, especially in renal impairment.

Other agents

These include drugs such as acarbose which reduce gut glucose absorption. Abdominal bloating commonly occurs with this drug.

Q11   Write short notes on the mode of action of drugs that lower blood pressure

Elevated blood pressure (BP) accelerates microvascular and macrovascular disease. Antihypertensive agents are widely prescribed. They include:

- **β-blockers** (e.g. atenolol):
  - the precise antihypertensive action of β-blockers is poorly understood
  - reduce cardiac output, alter baroreflex sensitivity and block peripheral adrenoreceptors
  - it is possible that their antihypertensive effect is central
- **α-blockers** (e.g. prazosin):
  - reduce BP by blocking post-synaptic α-receptors, causing vasodilatation
- **calcium channel blockers** (e.g. nifedipine):
  - act by blocking calcium influx through the slow transmembrane calcium channels
  - dihydropyridine calcium channel blockers such as nifedipine cause vasodilatation alone; non-dihydropyridine calcium channel blockers such as verapamil are also negative ionotropes
- **angiotensin-converting enzyme (ACE) inhibitors** (e.g. ramipril):
  - block the conversion of angiotensin I to angiotensin II
  - reduction in angiotensin II levels leads to reduced salt and water retention and vasodilatation
  - particularly useful in diabetic patients in whom they may protect against nephropathy
- **angiotensin II antagonists** (e.g. losartan):
  - used in those intolerant of ACE inhibitors, these drugs directly inhibit angiotensin II
  - actions are identical to ACE inhibitors
- **nitrates** (e.g. glyceryl trinitrate):
  - reduce blood pressure through a direct vasodilatating action on smooth muscle
- **central-acting antihypertensives** (e.g. methyldopa):
  - mode of action is uncertain.

Q12   Write short notes on the side effects of aminoglycosides

Aminoglycosides, such as gentamycin, neomycin and amikacin, are a class of **bactericidal** antibiotics, most effective against **aerobic Gram-negative** bacteria. They prevent bacterial protein synthesis by binding to bacterial ribosomes, which interferes with RNA binding and causes codon misreading.

Aminoglycosides are given intravenously, topically and intravitreally. Oral absorption is poor. Excretion is mainly via the **kidney**.

When aminoglycosides are given intravenously serum levels should be monitored to ensure therapeutic concentrations are reached and to prevent **nephrotoxicity** and **deafness**. Other side effects include loss of balance, tinnitus, nausea and vomiting. Rarely **myasthenia-like symptoms** occur; aminoglycosides should not be given to those with myasthenia gravis. Serious side effects are more common in the elderly and those with renal failure.

Topically, aminoglycosides cause **punctate keratitis**, **allergic conjuncti-vitis** and **contact dermatitis**. These are more common with neomycin. Conjunctival ischaemia has also been reported.

Retinal toxicity and necrosis have been reported with intravitreal use of aminoglycosides, particularly gentamycin. Amikacin is considered less retinotoxic.

Q13   What are the side effects of corticosteroids?

In addition to use as therapeutic replacement for **endocrine deficiency states**, corticosteroids are widely used to **modulate immune responses** (innate or adaptive). Corticosteroids affect both **tissue metabolism** (glucocorticoid actions) and **salt–water balance** (mineralocorticoid actions).

The collection of metabolic effects seen with extended treatment at higher doses is called **Cushing syndrome**. It is usually reversible on treatment withdrawal.

Adrenal suppression is a particularly important side effect of long-term steroid treatment. Any patient treated with systemic steroids for more than three weeks should be warned of the dangers of **sudden cessation**. To prevent this, all patients on long-term treatment should carry a **steroid treatment card** and doses must be **increased at times of stress and peri-operatively**.

The most commonly used corticosteroids in ophthalmic practice, dexamethasone and prednisolone, have only negligible and weak mineralocorticoid side effects, respectively.

Topical treatment maximises local steroid delivery with the minimum risk of systemic side effects. Important ocular side effects of topical treatment include **raised intraocular pressure**, occurring in up to 30%, and **reactivation of viral keratitis**.

Table 2 Side effects of corticosteroids

System	Side effect
General	<ul><li>Moon face</li><li>Buffalo hump</li><li>Central obesity (lemon on sticks)</li><li>Poor wound healing</li></ul>
Cardiovascular	<ul><li>Hypertension</li><li>Cardiomyopathy</li><li>Fragile veins, leading to easy bruising</li></ul>
Dermatological	<ul><li>Thinning of the skin</li><li>Acne</li><li>Striae</li></ul>
Gastrointestinal	<ul><li>Peptic ulceration</li></ul>
Endocrine	<ul><li>Reduced glucose tolerance</li><li>Secondary diabetes mellitus</li><li>Menstrual abnormalities</li></ul>
Renal	<ul><li>Water and sodium retention</li><li>Potassium wasting</li></ul>
Orthopaedic	<ul><li>Osteoporosis</li><li>Avascular necrosis of the femoral head</li><li>Premature epiphyseal closure, leading to stunted growth</li></ul>
Neurological/psychiatric	<ul><li>Proximal myopathy</li><li>Secondary benign intracranial hypertension</li><li>Labile mood/euphoria</li><li>Mania or depression</li></ul>
Haematological	<ul><li>Easy bruising</li><li>Increased susceptibility to infection</li><li>Apparent neutrophilia due to reduced neutrophil margination</li></ul>
Ophthalmological	<ul><li>Posterior subcapsular cataracts</li><li>Elevated intraocular pressure which may cause glaucoma</li><li>Reactivation of viral keratitis</li><li>Central serous chorioretinopathy</li></ul>

Q14 What are the current therapeutic strategies in the human immunodeficiency virus (HIV)?

Introduction

- HIV was recognised as the cause of acquired immunodeficiency syndrome (AIDS) in 1981.
- Treatment of HIV is fast-changing.
- Although cure is impossible, life expectancy of infected patients in the West is now many years.

Aims of treatment

- Reduction of mortality and morbidity.
- Suppression of viral load.
- Preservation and restoration of immune function.

When to treat

- Whenever symptomatic.
- Asymptomatic patients with less than 200 CD 4^+ T-cells/mm^3.
- Treatment of asymptomatic patients with higher CD 4^+ counts is controversial.

Classes of drugs

- **Protease inhibitors (PIs)**:
  - interfere with the protease enzyme that HIV uses to produce infectious viral particles.
- **Reverse transcriptase inhibitors** (RTIs) stop HIV replicating:
  - nucleoside RTIs (NRTIs) prevent reverse transcriptase from copying itself by providing it with faulty deoxyribonucleic acid (DNA) building blocks
  - non-nucleoside RTIs (NNRTIs) bind to and prevent the action of reverse transcriptase.

- **Fusion inhibitors**:
  - change the shape of HIV's gp41 envelope protein, preventing virus fusion and entry into host cells.

Treatment regimes

Highly active antiretroviral therapy (HAART) is the most effective treatment of HIV and involves the combination of two NRTIs with other agents:

- **NNRTI-based**: using a combination of one NNRTI and two NRTIs
- **PI-based**: one or two PI and two NRTIs
- **Triple NRTI**: appropriate when NNRTI or PI-based regimes are inappropriate.

Complications

- Drug interactions.
- Non-compliance.
- Resistance.
- Metabolic effects.

Q15   Write short notes comparing rods and cones

Table 3 compares structural features of rods and cones. Table 4 compares biochemical features of rods and cones. Table 5 compares functional/ organisational aspects of rods and cones.

Table 3   Comparison between structural features of rods and cones

	Rods	Cones
Number	• 92 million	• 5 million
Distribution	• Absent in the fovea • Highest density 15–20 degrees from the fovea	• Cone density highest in the fovea • BUT >90% cones outside the macula
Histology	• Larger nuclei with less heterochromatin	• Smaller nuclei with more heterochromatin
Ultrastructure (outer segments)	• Contain approx. 600–1000 discs • Longer and cylindrical • Same morphology across retina	• Invaginations of cytoplasmic membrane • Broader at the proximal end than at the apical end • Become smaller at the periphery
Ultrastructure (inner segments)	• More slender	• Wider
Synapses	• Triads: invaginations of rod bipolar cells with horizontal cell processes	• Invaginating synapses (with depolarising bipolar cells [ON-bipolar]) • Flat synapses (with hyperpolarising bipolar cells [OFF-bipolar])

Table 4 Comparison between biochemical aspects of rods and cones

	Rods	Cones
Chromophore	• 11-cis-retinal	• 11-cis-retinal
Opsin	• Rhodopsin	• 3 different types of opsins
Transduction cascade	• Both photoreceptor types use a similar transduction process	
Outer segment replacement	• Shed tips every morning	• Shed tips every evening
Neurotransmitter	• Glutamate	• Glutamate

Table 5 Comparison between functional/organisational aspects of rods and cones

	Rods	Cones
Colour vision	• Achromatic (peak sensitivity to 500 nm wavelength)	• Trichromatic (peak sensitivities at 437 nm, 533 nm and 564 nm for blue, green and red cones, respectively)
Illumination	• Greater sensitivity under scotopic conditions	• Greater sensitivity under photopic conditions
Convergence/ resolution	• Approximately 75 000 rods drive a single ganglion neuron • As a result, resolution (visual acuity) is lower	• In the fovea, single cones may drive single ganglion neurons • As a result, resolution (visual acuity) is superior
Temporal aspects	• Rods can respond to stimuli up to 20 Hz in theory, 6–10 Hz in practice • Temporal summation is present	• Cones can respond to higher stimulus frequencies
Response in bipolar cells	• Always sign-inversing to rod response	• Sign-inversing or sign-conserving
Pathways	• 4 neuron pathway to ganglion cell (rod–> bipolar cell–> rod amacrine (II) cell–> ganglion cell) • Mainly to magnocellular ganglion cells	• 3 neuron pathway to ganglion cell (cone–> bipolar cell–> ganglion cell) • Both to parvocellular and magnocellular ganglion cells

Q16   Describe the mechanisms regulating aqueous outflow

'Conventional' pathway

- 70–90% aqueous drains via the 'conventional' pathway.
- Aqueous passes from the anterior chamber to Schlemm's canal through the trabecular meshwork. Schlemm's canal is drained by aqueous veins which ultimately connect with the episcleral veins.
- Drainage is pressure dependent although the relationship is non-linear.
- Stimulation of β-receptors in the trabecular meshwork increases drainage.
- Miotics increase drainage by pulling on the scleral spur and 'opening up' the trabecular meshwork.
- All conditions which alter episcleral venous pressure affect intraocular pressure (IOP). Systemic antihypertensive agents reduce IOP; IOP rises in carotid cavernous fistulae.

'Non-conventional' pathway

- 10–30% aqueous drains via the 'non-conventional' or uveoscleral pathway.
- Aqueous passes through the intercellular spaces of the ciliary body into the suprachoroidal space and then across the sclera via the connective tissue sheaths surrounding the vessels and nerves that pierce it. Ultimately, aqueous passes into the vortex veins.
- This drainage route is independent of IOP.
- Prostaglandin $F_{2\alpha}$ analogues, such as latanoprost, increase uveoscleral drainage.

Q17   Describe the structures and relationships of different retinal ganglion cell types, including their connection to higher visual pathways

Ganglion cells are classified both anatomically and physiologically.

Anatomical classification

- Based on cell body size and dendritic morphology.
- α ganglion cells are large-bodied ganglion cells with broadly ramifying dendritic trees and large axons.
- β cells also have large cell bodies but more restricted dendritic arborisations.
- γ cells are those with small cell bodies and small axons.
- This anatomical classification correlates well with the physiological division of ganglion cells into W, X and Y classes.

Physiological classification

- The Y physiological class of ganglion cells corresponds to the α morphological class and exhibits non-linear spatial summation and responds briskly in a transient or phasic way.
- X cells correspond to β cells and have a shorter latency period and exhibit linear spatial summation. Their responses are usually sustained or tonic.
- W cells have large receptive fields, sluggish responses and slow response times. W physiological class correlates to γ cells, although this relationship is the weakest of the three.

Connections

- There are 10^6 ganglion cells in each eye and their axons form the optic nerve.
- Input to ganglion cells is from bipolar cells through which signals from the photoreceptors are transmitted.
- Neuronal interconnections at the retinal level cause most ganglion cells to have 'centre-surround' receptive fields.

- The vast majority of retinal ganglion cells project to the lateral geniculate nucleus (LGN) where they synapse with neurons that run to the primary visual cortex.
- The LGN is retinotopically mapped: layers 2, 3 and 5 receive ipsilateral input and layers 1, 4 and 6 contralateral input.
- Most α cells project to the magnocellular layers (1 and 2) and most β cells to the parvocellular layers (3–6).
- Some ganglion cells project to other midbrain nuclei: those running to the pretectal nuclei are involved in the pupillary light responses.

Q18   Write short notes on autoregulation of blood flow

Autoregulation is the process by which tissues and organs regulate their own blood supply and acts to keep blood flow constant in the face of varying supply or to adapt blood flow to local conditions. Autoregulation occurs in the kidneys, liver, myocardium, brain and skeletal muscle.

There are two main types of autoregulation:

- **myogenic autoregulation**:
  - most vascular beds have an intrinsic capacity to compensate for moderate changes in perfusion pressure by changing their vascular resistance so that blood flow remains relatively constant
  - this process is called myogenic autoregulation and is due to the intrinsic contractile response of vascular smooth muscle to stretch
  - myogenic autoregulation does not occur in the lungs
- **metabolic autoregulation**:
  - if tissue blood flow is inadequate, waste products such as potassium and hydrogen ions accumulate
  - metabolic autoregulation is the process by which such accumulation leads to localised vasodilatation
  - metabolic autoregulation is the main influence on coronary artery blood flow
  - metabolic autoregulation does not occur in the lungs: here a fall in oxygen concentration results in vasoconstriction.

Q19   Outline the differences between the sympathetic and parasympathetic branches of the autonomic nervous system

The sympathetic and parasympathetic branches of the autonomic nervous system have important anatomical, functional and pharmacological differences. These are outlined in Table 6 below.

Table 6   The autonomic nervous system

	Sympathetic	*Parasympathetic*
Function	'Fight or flight' (reduced peristalsis, tachycardia, pupillary dilation, bronchodilation)	'Rest and digest' (increased peristalsis, bradycardia, miosis, accommodation)
Origin	Spinal cord levels T1–L2	With cranial nerves III, VII, IX & X and from spinal cord levels S2–S4
Pre-ganglionic fibres	Both are myelinated. Nicotinic acetylcholine receptors are present in the ganglia. Parasympathetic fibres are longer	
Ganglia	Near to origin, mostly paravertebral	Near to target organ
Post-ganglionic fibres	Both are non-myelinated type C fibres. Sympathetic fibres are longer	
Target organ synapse	Noradrenaline is the transmitter (exception: acetylcholine in sweat glands). α- and β-adrenoreceptors present	Muscarinic cholinergic receptors

Q20   Write short notes on steroid receptors. Illustrate your answer with reference to the glucocorticoid receptor

- The steroid receptor superfamily includes receptors for steroid hormones (mineralocorticoids, glucocorticoids and sex hormones), thyroid hormones, retinoids and vitamin D.
- These compounds differ greatly from each other in chemical structure and function but are all small hydrophobic molecules with similar modes of action.
- The glucocorticoid receptor is a typical steroid receptor:
  - there is only a single class of glucocorticoid receptor and it is found in nearly all cells
  - like all steroid receptors it is intracellular
  - glucocorticoids must diffuse across the plasma membrane before combining with and activating the receptor
  - heat shock protein (hsp)-90 is associated with the glucocorticoid receptor and acts as a molecular chaperone, maintaining the unactivated receptor in its optimum configuration and preventing the unbound receptor from migrating to the nucleus
  - following cortisol binding, hsp-90 detaches from the receptor and the receptor–ligand complex migrates to the nucleus
  - in the nucleus the receptor–ligand complex binds to DNA at promoter regions of steroid-responsive target genes, inducing or suppressing their transcription
  - there are between 10 and 100 steroid-responsive genes in each cell: this explains the wide range of action of steroids.

Q21   Describe the physiological and pharmacological mechanisms involved in water transfer through tissue

Overview

- The human body consists of about two-thirds water by weight.
- Control of the distribution of this water is important for well-being and manipulation of its distribution can be important clinically.
- Body fluid is divided between the intravascular, interstitial and intracellular compartments:
  - the intravascular and intracellular compartments do not communicate directly but are linked by the interstitial compartment.
- Transfer between compartments is a passive process due to the balance of hydrostatic and osmotic pressures across the separating membrane.
- When water is described as being 'pumped' between compartments, it is not water but solutes which are pumped: this creates a concentration gradient down which water transfers by osmosis.

Hydrostatic pressure

- This is elevated in many conditions such as heart failure. Such conditions lead to the formation of dependent oedema.
- Treatment with diuretics reduces intravascular volume, favouring fluid resorption by reducing hydrostatic pressure.

Osmotic pressure

- Although water can cross plasma membranes relatively easily, differences in osmotic pressure between compartments result from the relative impermeability of the plasma membrane to ions.
- Transmembrane ion concentration differences result from metabolic activity, active pumps and secondary active pump mechanisms.
- Many drug actions are due to osmotic fluid shift:
  - osmotic diuretics like mannitol draw fluid from the interstitial compartment into the intravascular space and are useful in treating conditions such as cerebral oedema

- most other diuretics act by altering ion transport across the nephron, usually by blocking specific ion channels or pumps. For example, loop diuretics reduce Na/Cl/K co-transport in the thick ascending limb of the loop of Henle
- carbonic anhydrase catalyses the reversible reaction $CO_2 + H_2O \leftrightarrow HCOO_3^- + H^+$ and inhibition of this enzyme reduces aqueous humour secretion by altering ion distribution across the ciliary epithelium
- hypertonic tear solutions are used to reduce corneal oedema by creating an osmotic gradient down which fluid passes from the cornea
- ouabain inhibits the Na/K–ATPase pump: when applied to the cornea *in vitro* this causes stromal oedema due to failure of the 'endothelial pump' mechanism.

Q22   Write short notes on endocytosis. Illustrate your answer with an example from the eye

Overview

Endocytosis is a form of transmembrane transport by which molecules cross inwards through cellular membranes in vesicles. Most macromolecules too large to enter cells by diffusion enter by endocytosis. Uptake of cellular material by endocytosis is called phagocytosis; pinocytosis is endocytosis of fluid.

Mechanism

Endocytosis is an active process requiring energy. It involves invagination of localised areas of the plasma membrane which then pinch off to form vesicles within the cell. Often these vesicles are destined for intracellular lysozomes. The plasma membrane components are continually returned to the cell surface in an endocytotic–exocytotic cycle.

In the process of receptor-mediated endocytosis, cell surface receptors that bind specific molecules become internalised in clathrin-coated pits. Following absorption, the clathrin-coated pits are internalised into intracellular vesicles which fuse with endosomes leading to degradation of the contents.

Endocytosis in the eye

Shed portions of the tips of photoreceptor outer segments are taken up by phagocytosis and digested by the retinal pigment epithelium (RPE). This process has a diurnal rhythm with rod tips being shed maximally 1 hour after the onset of light and cone tips 2–3 hours after the onset of darkness. In rods, RPE cells are thought to have specific receptors for rod outer segments at their apices and these segments are absorbed in clathrin-coated pits. The signal for shedding is thought to originate from within the retina and the process involves second messengers, possibly cAMP. Digestion of the phagocytosed rod tips is aided by the numerous lysozomal acid hydrolases found within the RPE and certain components are 'recycled', being passed back to the photoreceptors.

Q23   Discuss mechanisms by which bacteria destroy tissue

Bacteria destroy tissue by direct and indirect means.

Direct

- Specific toxins fall into two classes: endotoxins and exotoxins:
  - **endotoxins** are lipopolysaccharides which, although antigenically distinct, have similar core structures. Their main cause of tissue damage is by complement activation. Endotoxins also cause fever and shock. All Gram-negative bacteria produce endotoxins
  - **exotoxins** are proteins produced by certain Gram-positive bacteria. They are heat-labile and highly antigenic. Examples include the neurotoxin of *Clostridium tetani*. Exotoxins are able to cause tissue damage at sites distant from the primary infection site.
- Many bacteria produce **enzymes** which cause local tissue injury and facilitate their spread. These include:
  - collagenase: from bacilli, disrupts collagen in connective tissue
  - coagulase: facilitates fibrin deposition and coagulates plasma
  - hyaluronidase: hydrolyses hyaluronic acid in the extracellular matrix of connective tissue
  - streptokinase: most often produced by haemolytic streptococci, activates fibrinolysin and dissolves clots
  - leukocidins: certain bacteria such as group A haemolytic streptococci produce enzymes such as streptolysin O which lyse red blood cells and tissue cells.

Indirect

- Immune activation is essential for combating bacterial infection but an excessive or inappropriate response, called a **hypersensitivity response**, will lead to tissue damage. An example is the cell-mediated type IV hypersensitivity reaction that occurs with *Mycobacterium tuberculosis* infection.

Q24   List the ophthalmic manifestations of the acquired immunodeficiency syndrome (AIDS)

Anterior segment

- Increased eyelash length.
- Episcleritis.
- Keratitis.
- Uveitis.

Posterior segment

- Retinal oedema and haemorrhages.
- Microaneurysms.
- Cotton wool spots.
- Retinal vascular sheathing.
- Choroidal granulomata.
- Progressive outer retinal necrosis (PORN).
- Papillitis.

Opportunistic infections

- Bacterial:
  - syphilitic chorioretinitis
  - *Pneumocystis carinii* retinitis.
- Viral:
  - cytomegalovirus retinitis:
    - (i)   unifocal or mulitfocal 'pizza pie' retinopathy
    - (ii) necrotising retinitis
    - (iii) retinal vasculitis
    - (iv) rhegmatogenous retinal detachment following atrophic hole formation.
- Protozoal:
  - *Toxoplasma* retinochoroiditis.

Neoplastic

- Kaposi sarcoma:
  - skin
  - conjunctival.
- Lymphoma:
  - primary intraocular
  - adnexal.

Q25 List the clinical manifestations of giant cell arteritis

Giant cell arteritis (GCA) is a non-immunological multisystem vasculitis which preferentially involves medium and large arteries of the head and neck. GCA occurs in all races but is commonest in Caucasians. GCA is more common in women and rare before 50 years. The erythrocyte sedimentation rate is usually elevated and temporal artery biopsy may be performed for diagnosis.

Clinical features include:

- **systemic**:
  - weight loss
  - malaise
  - anorexia
  - fatigue
  - fever
  - polymyalgia rheumatica with proximal limb girdle pain and weakness
  - rarely aortitis, myocardial infarction or cerebral infarction
- **local**:
  - tenderness over the temporal artery
  - loss of temporal artery pulsation
  - temporal artery thickening
  - jaw claudication
- **ocular**:
  - central or branch retinal artery occlusion
  - anterior segment ischaemia
  - choroidal infarction
- **neuro-ophthalmic**:
  - arteritic ischaemic optic neuropathy following involvement of the posterior ciliary arteries
  - oculomotor palsies are caused by muscle or nerve ischaemia
  - cortical blindness.

Q26   Discuss the pathological effects of ionising radiation

Ionising radiation exists as both electromagnetic radiation and free particles. External beam radiotherapy is used to treat many malignant tumours of the head and neck, including ocular tumours such as retinoblastoma and melanoma. Choroidal melanomas can be treated by brachytherapy, in which a gamma ray emitter is applied to the sclera overlying the tumour.

Although ionising radiation can cause direct tissue injury, its major mechanism of damage is secondary to free radical formation. The pathological effects of ionising radiation are dose related.

Acute effects

Ionising radiation causes acute tissue injury by damaging deoxyribonucleic acid (DNA), resulting in defective mitosis, and through vascular damage after endothelial injury. The acute effects of ionising radiation are more marked in rapidly dividing tissues.

Commonly, effects include:

- gut – **diarrhoea** (intestinal epithelial loss)
- skin – **desquamation** and **hair loss**
- eye – **superficial keratitis**
- bone marrow – **suspension of cell renewal** (granulocytes before erythrocytes)
- gonads – increased risk of **malformations** and **stillbirth**.

With very high exposures massive necrosis of normal tissues occurs.

Chronic effects

As well as **increased risk of malignancy**, due to DNA damage, **atrophy** and **fibrosis** may develop. This is partly due to reduced cell renewal and partly due to development of an endarteritis obliterans, probably caused by endothelial injury. Fibrosis may lead to **restrictive lung disease** and **intestinal strictures**. **Fertility** may be reduced. **Cataracts** can develop. Fibrosis of glandular tissues causes **dry eyes and mouth**. **Radiation retinopathy** occurs when endothelial damage allows leakage of plasma constituents into the surrounding tissues.

Q27   Draw a diagram of the normal retinal capillary. How is the structure altered in diabetes?

In diabetic capillaries:

- structural changes lead to both **occlusion** of and **leakage** from capillaries
- basement membranes become **homogeneously thickened**
- endothelial cell damage and proliferation result in **intimal fibrosis** and vessel narrowing
- this is compounded by **changes in red blood cells** which cause defective oxygen transport and an increase in the stickiness and aggregation of platelets
- despite being thickened the basement membranes of diabetic subjects are **abnormally leaky**, probably due to **loss of pericytes**, and there is increased passive transudation of plasma proteins into the surrounding tissue
- it is thought that this leakage is due to loss of pericytes which are normally involved in the maintenance of endothelial barrier function
- normally there is about one pericyte per endothelial cell but this ratio falls in diabetes
- the protein transudate triggers a fibrous and vascular response
- **proteinuria** is the first indication of diabetic kidney disease
- changes in basement membrane structure are thought to be responsible for the peripheral neuropathy, nephropathy and retinopathy of diabetes.

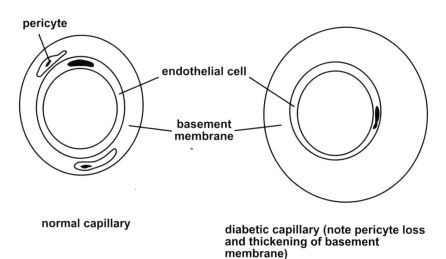

Figure 2   Cross-sections through a normal and a diabetic capillary.

Q28   Write short notes on the pathogenesis of atheromatous plaques

Atherosclerosis is the most common disorder leading to death and morbidity in the western world. More people are killed by atherosclerosis than by all forms of cancer combined. Although any artery can be affected, atherosclerosis is most common in large- and medium-sized arteries.

Risk factors

Risk factors include:

● male sex
● increasing age
● diabetes
● smoking
● hypertension
● dyslipidaemia.

It is not known whether atherosclerotic plaques develop from fatty streaks. Evidence against this includes their different topographical distributions and different cholesterol : triglyceride ratios. There is no evidence of an immunological basis to the development of atherosclerosis.

Pathogenesis

● Endothelial damage is believed to be the primary step in plaque formation.
● Platelets then adhere to the injured endothelium and stimulate endothelial smooth muscle proliferation by release of platelet-derived growth factor.
● Intra- and extracellular lipid accumulation follows loss of endothelial cell barrier function.
● Lipid-laden macrophages and other inflammatory cells are often seen.
● These changes cause the intima to thicken.

Sequelae

● Plaque growth and luminal narrowing.
● Thinning of the adventitia media and aneurysm formation.

- Plaque fissure:
    - platelet microthrombi form if this is small
    - if large, potentially occlusive or embolic thrombi occur.
- Intraplaque haemorrhage is common.

Atherosclerotic plaques are not thought to regress.

Q29   Describe the causes and effects of ulcers

An ulcer is a **discontinuity in an epithelial-lined surface caused by the sloughing of necrotic inflammatory material.** Ulcers occur on all epithelial-covered tissues, including the cornea, gut and skin.

All causes of acute inflammation cause tissue ulceration:

- **trauma**
- **infection**:
  - bacterial, e.g. *Pseudomonas* keratitis
  - viral, e.g. dendritic ulcers due to herpes simplex type 1 virus
  - fungal
  - amoebic, e.g. *Acanthamoeba* keratitis
- **immunological**:
  - granuloma formation such as in tuberculosis or syphilis
  - peripheral corneal ulceration in vasculitides such as Wegener's granulomatosis
- **hypersensitivity**:
  - marginal corneal ulcers are a response to lid margin staphylococcal exotoxins
- **chemical**
- **ischaemia**:
  - arterial, as in Raynaud's syndrome
  - venous, as occurs as a post-thrombotic phenomenon
- **neurotrophic**:
  - occur in the cornea following herpes zoster infection
- **radiation**.

The natural history of ulcers includes:

- **repair** with return to normal epithelial and underlying structure
- **regeneration** and formation of scar tissue which may contract:
  - corneal scars are less organised and more opaque than the normal cornea and may reduce visual acuity as well as cause surface irregularity
  - duodenal ulcers cause pyloric stenosis
- **invasion** of underlying structures:
  - when corneal ulceration extends through the full thickness of the stroma, intraocular pressure causes Descemet's membrane to bulge out. This is known as a descemetocele

   – further thinning can result in corneal perforation which may be plugged by prolapsed iris tissue. If this iris tissue epithelialises an anterior staphyloma results

   – gastric ulcers cause haemorrhage by invading underlying blood vessels

- **chronic persisting inflammation** and ulceration:

   – commonly corneal vascularisation results

- **malignant change**:

   – Marjolin's skin ulcers (usually venous)

   – gastric ulcers.

Q30   What are free radicals? Write short notes explaining why retinal photoreceptors are particularly vulnerable to free radicals

A free radical is an **atom or molecule with at least one unpaired electron**. This property makes free radicals **highly reactive** towards other molecular species. They are produced:

- as a **normal product of oxidative phosphorylation**
- by **enzymatic systems** (e.g. during the enzymatic synthesis of prostaglandins, NADPH [nicotinamide adenine dinucleotide phosphate] oxidase system of phagocytes)
- by non-enzymatic oxidation catalysed by **iron or catalytic metals** such as copper
- by **ionising radiation**
- by **photo-oxidation** (e.g. ultraviolet [UV] light)
- by **auto-oxidation of lipids**.

Several features of retinal photoreceptors make them particularly vulnerable to damage from free radicals:

- the membrane of the photoreceptor outer segment has a **high proportion of highly polyunsaturated fatty acids**. Polyunsaturated fatty acids are sensitive to peroxidation in proportion to the number of double bonds
- the rod inner segment is very **rich in mitochondria**, which inevitably produce free radicals
- the **choroid circulation** provides an **excellent oxygen supply** which elevates the risk of oxidative damage
- vertebrate retinas maintained *in vitro* have the **highest rate of oxygen consumption per milligram of protein** of any body tissue except the adrenal gland
- the retina is **exposed to UV light and blue light** in children and adolescents despite some filtering by the cornea and absorption by the high ascorbate concentrations in the aqueous. The retina is exposed to blue light and some UV light in pseudophakic individuals.

Free radical mediated damage has been implicated in the pathogenesis of age-related macular degeneration.

Q31   Describe ways in which cells die

The mechanism of cell death is usually determined by the insult causing it.

- **Apoptosis** is the process of genetically programmed cell death. Expression of a particular 'apoptosis gene' leads to cytoplasmic and nuclear shrinking, and nucleic acid degradation by calcium- and magnesium-dependent endonucleases before cell digestion by lysozymes from adjacent cells. No inflammatory response occurs. Apoptosis may be triggered by genes such as p53 in damaged cells or may occur as part of normal development, as happens during the formation of the normal web spaces between digits.
- Death by **cell lysis** commonly follows viral infection but may also follow osmotic shock.
- Various drugs kill cells by **disrupting metabolic pathways**. Bacteriocidal antibiotics such as penicillins, which inhibit cell wall synthesis, and aminoglycosides, which are inhibitors of protein synthesis, act in this way as do many chemotherapeutic agents used in cancer treatment.
- Other drugs kill cells by **blocking respiratory pathways**, leading to an inability to maintain metabolism. An example is cyanide: this blocks reduction of molecular oxygen by inhibiting cytochrome oxidase.
- **Essential nutrient supply** may be interrupted. This occurs after central retinal artery occlusion where ischaemia leads to rapid death of the inner retinal areas.

Q32   Write short notes on viral replication

Viruses are acellular and **unable to replicate independently**, instead needing to enter a cell to replicate.

Viruses comprise genetic material enclosed in a protein shell, the capsid, made up of identical subunits. Viral genomes may be coded for by either deoxyribonucleic acid (DNA) or ribonucleic acid (RNA).

There are several stages to viral replication:

- **attachment** to host cell by random collision, electrostatic attachment or by specific host receptors. This process is called **adsorption**
- cell **penetration** occurs either by viropexis or by fusion of the viral envelope and the cell membrane
- host cell enzymes **digest** the capsid
- nucleic acid **replication** occurs (see below)
- **assembly** of the newly replicated virion occurs
- a period of **maturation** follows
- newly formed virus particles are **released** by cell lysis or budding through the cell membrane.

Nucleic acid replication differs with nucleic acid type. DNA viruses, with the exception of parvovirus, replicate in the cell nucleus using host cell enzymes. No host enzymes exist for copying RNA from RNA and so RNA viruses must replicate in the cytoplasm. There are several ways this can occur, for example using reverse transcriptase to make DNA from an RNA template from which a complementary RNA sequence can then be made.

Q33   Contrast Gram-negative and Gram-positive bacteria

Bacteria are classified as Gram-positive or Gram-negative according to their microscopic appearance following Gram staining. Gram staining reflects cell wall structure.

Table 7   Gram-positive and Gram-negative bacteria

	Gram-positive	*Gram-negative*
Appearance on Gram stain	Blue	Red
Cell wall structure	Simple. Approximately 50% peptidoglycan and 40–45% acidic polymer	Complex. Thin layer of peptidoglycan (5%) and an outer layer made up of proteins, phospolipids and lipopolysaccharides
Toxins produced	Not all produce toxins. Those that do produce heat-labile exotoxins which are proteins, usually enzymes, and not derived from the cell wall. Exotoxins have specific pharmacological actions	All produce endotoxins which are derived from lipopolysaccharides within the cell wall. These are heat-labile, strongly antigenic and generally more potent than exotoxins. Endotoxins have non-specific inflammatory actions
Susceptibility to antibiotics	The cell wall of Gram-positive bacteria is polar and carries a negative charge, influencing the penetration of ionised molecules. Most antibiotics carry a positive charge and penetrate well	Their complex cell wall structure makes Gram-negative bacteria less susceptible to antibiotics

Q34   Describe the chief mechanisms by which bacteria acquire resistance to antibiotics

Bacterial resistance to antibiotics invariably follows genetic change in the bacteria which may be due either to random mutation or to transfer of genetic material from other bacteria which themselves are already antibiotic resistant.

Gene mutation

- Single-point mutations occur in *Escherichia coli* every 10^5–10^7 divisions.
- Gene mutation is an important cause of resistance to antituberculous drugs such as rifampicin.

Genetic transfer

- Extrachromosomal DNA, in the form plasmids, can be passed between unrelated bacteria when direct contact occurs. This is called **conjugation** and involves transfer of large amounts of genetic material.
- Chromosomal deoxyribonucleic acid (DNA) can pass between bacteria either directly ('**transformation**') or in a bacteriophage virus ('**transduction**'). Before the transferred genetic material can become effective it has to be incorporated into the host chromosomal DNA, which must therefore be similar in structure to the donor chromosomal DNA. Transformation is the least clinically important mechanism of acquired bacterial antibiotic resistance.

Bacteria become resistant to antibiotics by:

- destroying or inactivating the antibiotic (e.g. acetylation of aminoglycosides)
- excluding the antibiotic
- modifying the antibiotic's target site (e.g. when erythromycin fails to bind ribosomes)
- using alternative enzyme pathways that are resistant to the drug (e.g. enzymes resistant to sulphonamides and trimethoprim).

Q35   Discuss the microbiology of *Pseudomonas aeruginosa*

Pseudomonas aeruginosa is a **strictly aerobic, oxidase-positive, non-motile rod** which is subtyped by bacteriophage typing. It is a virulent ocular pathogen due to the **copious amounts of enzymes** it produces. These cause tissue damage and, via the action of β-lactamase, render many antibiotics ineffective. Additionally, all *Pseudomonas* species produce a water-soluble pigment, pyocin, that diffuses through growth media. Different strains produce different pyocins.

Pseudomonas species appear to be **dependent on iron for growth** and changes in iron metabolism affect their virulence. *Pseudomonas* species are **incapable of penetrating healthy corneal epithelium** well but in those with epithelial defects *Pseudomonas aeruginosa* can cause a devastating **keratitis**, capable of perforating the cornea within 24 hours in extreme cases. **Contact lens wearers** are at a far greater risk of *Pseudomonas* keratitis because corneal epithelial trauma is almost inevitable with their use. Thermal burns, vitamin A deficiency and immunosuppression all predispose to pseudomonal corneal infection. *Pseudomonas* species can cause endophthalmitis.

Fluoroquinolone antibiotics such as ofloxacin are usually effective monotherapy in the treatment of *Pseudomonas aeruginosa* infections.

Outside the eye, *Pseudomonas aeruginosa* frequently **colonises the lungs** of those with chronic airways disease. *Pseudomonas* species also cause **urinary tract** and **wound infections**.

Q36   What precautions would be taken to prevent spread of methicillin-resistant *Staphylococcus aureus* (MRSA) infection from patient to patient on an ophthalmic ward?

MRSA is a relatively common nosocomial pathogen which is resistant to many commonly used antibiotics. The main route of MRSA transmission between hospital patients is on the hands of health workers. Infected patients are the main reservoir of MRSA but health workers themselves, medical equipment and environmental surfaces can also act as reservoirs.

Standard precautions are those which should be observed when examining all patients. If a patient is known or suspected to be MRSA positive, additional contact precautions are necessary.

Standard precautions

- **Hand washing** is by far the most important single precaution shown to prevent MRSA spread. Hands should be washed before and after each episode of patient contact. Washing may even be necessary between tasks on the same patient to prevent cross infection. Hand washing should be performed after contact with medical equipment and bodily fluids. Hand washing is necessary even when gloves are worn.
- **Gloves** should be donned in all cases when there may be contact with blood, mucous membranes or body fluids. Gloves should be disposed of appropriately as soon as the patient encounter has finished.
- When splashes of body fluids are likely, **masks** and **gowns** should be worn.
- **Equipment** should be cleaned appropriately between patients.
- Soiled **laundry** should be handled with due care.
- Patient rooms, toilets and other frequently touched surfaces should be **cleaned daily**.

Contact precautions

Patients with known or suspected MRSA should be kept in **isolation** or in an area with other infected patients. As much as is reasonable, their **movement**

should be restricted. During patient contact gloves must always be worn. **Gowns** must be put on if substantial patient contact is anticipated. Whenever possible, **dedicated equipment** should be allocated for use on single or cohorts of MRSA-positive patients.

Q37   Write short notes on the principles of sterilisation

Sterilisation is the destruction of all microbial life, including highly resistant bacterial endospores, using a chemical or physical process. Disinfection is a less thorough procedure and involves the removal of most, but not all, microbial life. Chemical germicides are usually used as disinfectants.

   In hospital, the major sterilisation techniques used include:

- **moist heat** by steam autoclaving. Spores take the longest time to kill and the time taken is temperature and pressure dependent. This technique is suitable for sterilising most heat-resistant surgical instruments
- **dry heat** via a hot air oven. This relies on conduction of heat rather than heat transfer through condensation. It requires higher temperatures and longer times than moist heat and so is not appropriate for heat-sensitive materials
- **ethylene oxide gas** sterilises at 55°C and so can be used to sterilise heat-sensitive instruments. The gas is toxic by contact and explosive
- **irradiation** is used to sterilise many single-use products such as syringes
- **chemical germicides** are used to sterilise heat-sensitive instruments.

Reusable heat-stable instruments that enter the bloodstream or normally sterile tissues should be sterilised using heat-based techniques.

Q38   Compare and contrast bacteria, viruses and chlamydia

Bacteria, viruses and chlamydia are all important ocular pathogens. An understanding of their similarities and differences helps us understand the mechanism and pattern of disease that they cause as well as the way that they are treated.

Table 8   Comparison of bacteria, viruses and chlamydia

	Bacteria	Viruses	Chlamydia
Overview	Lack distinct nuclear membrane (prokaryotic)	The simplest form of life known, consisting of a protein capsule containing a genetic code	Originally classified as viruses, chlamydia are now known to be Gram-negative non-motile coccoid bacteria
Size	Can be seen under light microscope	10–100 times smaller than bacteria, meaning that most cannot be seen by light microscope	Can be seen under light microscope
Nucleic acid	Both deoxyribonucleic acid (DNA) and ribonucleic acid (RNA)	Either DNA or RNA	Both DNA and RNA
Metabolism	Independent	None; viruses are inert outside host cells	Incapable of energy metabolism and lacking in many biosynthetic pathways
Replication	By binary fission	Must enter host cell to multiply	Chlamydia need to enter a host cell before they can multiply
Treatment	Antibiotics generally effective	Antiviral agents are only effective against certain viral infections	Antibiotics generally effective
Vaccination	Yes, for some	Yes, for some	No

Q39   Write short notes on genetic linkage analysis. Give an example

Background

- During meiosis, crossing over and exchange of segments can occur at any point along the length of homologous chromosomes.
- When two genes lie on the same chromosome, the closer they are together the less likely a crossing over is to occur and the more likely they are to be transmitted together.
- Gene loci are said to be linked if the two alleles do not show independent segregation in meiosis.

Clinical importance

Genetic linkage studies are used clinically to assess the likelihood of a subject having a condition, which itself may not be readily detectable at that time, based on the presence or absence of a readily identifiable trait.

Method

- Genetic linkage is established using laboratory techniques such as *in situ* hybridisation or by family or pedigree analysis.
- For pedigree analysis large pedigrees are needed and all those with the disease must have the same gene causing the condition.

Example

In one of the earliest genetic linkage studies, a British family with congenital cataract (Coppock cataract) had their condition linked to the Duffy blood group found on chromosome 1.

Q40   Discuss the genetic mechanisms involved in neoplasia

Overview

- Almost by definition, all tumours are genetically abnormal in some way. This accounts for their autonomous and abnormal proliferative capacity.
- Genetic abnormalities are either inherited or acquired.

Mechanism

- Inherited genetic abnormalities account for about 10% of tumours:
  - these may predispose to a particular tumour:
    - (i)   mutation of the retinoblastoma gene on chromosome 12 causes retinoblastoma
  - or, if a gene is involved in control of apoptosis or nucleic acid repair, to a wide variety of tumours:
    - (i)   the high incidence of ultraviolet light-related skin cancers in xeroderma pigmentosa is due to defective deoxyribonucleic acid (DNA) repair
    - (ii)   in the Li–Fraumeni syndrome there is a defect in the p53 tumour suppresser gene normally involved in control of apoptosis
  - some tumours are inherited in a multifactorial manner.
- Acquired genetic abnormalities have many causes:
  - random mutation
  - ultraviolet radiation
  - ionising radiation
  - viral infection
  - carcinogen exposure.

Mechanism

There are three main ways in which genetic abnormalities cause neoplasia:

- activation of an oncogene:
  - oncogenes are overexpressed or amplified genes whose products code for factors involved in cell growth or differentiation

- oncogenes have a dominant effect at the cellular level
- the *ras* oncogene is present in 90% of pancreatic cancers
- alteration in the gene regulation of apoptosis:
  - this leads to increased cell survival
  - *bcl*-2 gene activation prevents apoptosis
- inactivation of tumour suppression genes:
  - tumour suppressor genes are recessive at the cellular level
  - inactivation of the tumour suppressor gene p53, which regulates nuclear transcription, is the most common genetic abnormality in neoplasms.

Q41   Write short notes on prenatal testing

- Prenatal testing is used to assess the likelihood of a fetus having a specific structural or genetic abnormality before it is born.
- Early in the second trimester **abdominal echography** may be performed to look for structural abnormalities (e.g. of the heart). From about the same time maternal blood α-fetoprotein levels can be measured and, if raised, may suggest a fetal neural tube defect.
- At approximately 9–12 weeks' gestation **chorionic villus sampling** (CVS) can be performed. CVS is particularly suited for genetic analysis of inherited disease such as translocations, enzymopathies and single gene defects.
- **Amniocentesis** is carried out from about 16 weeks and the fluid obtained used for cytologic, biochemic and cytogenic assays.
- From around 18 weeks **fetal blood sampling** from the umbilical cord may be attempted. This is particularly useful when CVS, amniocentesis or ultrasound findings are equivocal and rapid chromosome analysis is necessary.
- **Fetoscopy** is more invasive still and is used for direct inspection of the fetus and for umbilical cord blood sampling.
- Invasive tests such as fetoscopy, fetal blood sampling, amniocentesis and CVS all have an associated risk of miscarriage.

Q42   Write short notes on the polymerase chain reaction

Background

- The polymerase chain reaction (PCR) is a laboratory technique by which a single strand of deoxyribonucleic acid (DNA) can be amplified a million times in 20 cycles.
- PCR requires less than 1% of genomic DNA needed for Southern or Northern blotting and is a faster, easier, cheaper and more sensitive technique.
- To use PCR the exact sequences of nucleotides which flank the DNA region of interest must be known, although the sequence itself need not be known.
- Because the flanking sequences of so many genes are known it is possible to use PCR to identify differences between organisms.
- Amplified DNA can also be used to identify criminal suspects or disease-causing viruses.

Method

- PCR involves mixing target DNA, two oligonucleotide primers with sequences that are complementary to the region of target DNA flanking the area of interest, a heat-stable DNA polymerase and a pool of nucleotides.
- The mixture is heated to just below $100°C$, denaturing the target DNA into single strands. The mixture is allowed to cool and the primers hybridise to opposite strands of the target sequence.
- Next, DNA polymerase initiates synthesis of two complementary strands of DNA, each an exact replica of the original target sequence.
- The cycle is then repeated further, amplifying the target sequence.
- It is possible to amplify ribonucleic acid (RNA) using PCR. Reverse transcriptase must first be used to produce a complementary DNA sequence to the target RNA. PCR primers are then added to the mixture, together with DNA polymerase, producing a double-stranded DNA molecule which is then amplified using the techniques outlined above.

Q43   What is a chromosomal translocation? Illustrate your answer with an example associated with ocular disease

Chromosomal translocations are **structural chromosomal abnormalities that result when two non-homologous chromosomes break and then reunite with the segments that broke off being exchanged**.

In most cases there is no loss of genetic material during chromosomal translocation. Karyotype studies have shown that one in 500 individuals are normal translocation carriers.

Sometimes people who appear to be balanced translocation carriers by karyotype analysis may be clinically abnormal: this happens when the break in the chromosome occurs in the middle of a gene, leading to formation of an abnormal non-functional protein product.

A **Robertsonian translocation** occurs when two acrocentric chromosomes break near their centromeres and fuse together with loss of their short arms. Although this gives a karyotype of 45 chromosomes, the phenotype is unaffected because the short arms of acrocentric chromosomes all contain multiple copies of genes coding for ribosomal ribonucleic acid (RNA). However, the progeny of such karyotypes may be affected as they can end up with three gene copies due to the effect of the translocation.

Ocular features of Down syndrome include strabismus, blepharitis, keratoconus, cataract and myopia. Down syndrome is most commonly due to trisomy 21 but may also be caused by a Robertsonian translocation of chromosome 21.

Q44   Describe the causes and effects of occlusive disease occurring in muscular arteries and arterioles

Muscular arteries include the renal and cerebral arteries and are branches of elastic arteries such as the aorta and carotid arteries. Arterioles are the smallest of arterial vessels. The causes and effects of arterial and arteriolar occlusion are described below.

Causes

- **Atherosclerosis** is a proliferative endothelial disease which most frequently involves medium- and large-sized arteries. Endothelial injury leads to platelet adhesion to the damaged area and subsequent release of platelet-derived growth factor causes intimal smooth muscle proliferation. Loss of endothelial barrier function results in intra- and extracellular lipid accumulation. Occlusion may occur gradually as the plaque increases in size or abruptly if the plaque ruptures, triggering thrombosis. Atherosclerosis is very common and is the leading cause of death in the developed world.
- **Thrombi** are solid plugs formed from the components of the blood. In high-flow systems such as arteries the trigger for thrombus formation is changes in the vessel wall, such as following atherosclerotic plaque rupture. Microscopically, thrombi comprise a clotted mesh of fibrin and platelets firmly attached to the vessel wall.
- An **embolus** is an abnormal mass of solid, liquid or gas carried in the bloodstream from one site to impact in a vessel elsewhere. 99% of occlusive emboli are detached thrombi but other causes include air (following trauma to the great vessels of the neck), nitrogen (in divers), fat (following fractures), amniotic fluid (as an obstetric complication), infection or tumour. Occlusive emboli most commonly occur in the lower limbs. Microscopically, the appearance of emboli reflects their constituents.
- **Vasculitides** are a diverse range of inflammatory disorders:
  - under the light microscope a dense infiltrate of acute and chronic inflammatory cells is seen in **immunologically-mediated** vasculitides such as Wegener's disease. Special immunological techniques usually demonstrate abnormal depositions of immunoglobulin and complement in the intima and media

— giant cell arteritis (GCA) is an example of an **idiopathic** vasculitis. GCA affects medium- and large-sized arteries and most frequently involves arteries of the head and neck. In up to 50% it is associated with polymyalgia rheumatica. Microscopically, intimal thickening and oedema are seen together with a dense chronic inflammatory and giant cell reaction with phagocytosis of fragmented elastic fibres.

- **Vasospasm** tends to affect distal vessels and is seen in Raynaud's phenomenon.
- **External compression** can result from trauma, tourniquets or orthopaedic casts. Supracondylar fractures of the femur obstruct the popliteal artery when the distal fragment is displaced posteriorly.

Effects

Acute obstruction of an end artery to an organ with high metabolic demands leads to tissue damage and organ failure within minutes. For example, ischaemic stroke rapidly follows cerebral artery occlusion.

More gradual occlusion of an artery may allow development of collateral vessels. In this situation symptoms of organ dysfunction may only occur when metabolic demand rises, such as in exertional angina, or when occlusion reaches a critical point.

An important complication of retinal vascular occlusion is neovascularisation. Although more common after venous than arterial occlusion, this can lead to tractional retinal detachment and vitreous haemorrhage.

Q45   List the major roles of complement

The complement cascade is a series of about 26 **heat-labile plasma proteins** which are capable of combining with antibodies on cell surfaces and which form an integral component of the **inflammatory response** as well as both the innate and adaptive **immune responses**.

Functions include:

- **opsonisation** (e.g. by C3b), the process of making micro-organisms more susceptible to phagocytosis by 'labelling' them
- mediating **antibody-dependent cytolysis** by polymerising on cell surfaces to form pores in the cell membrane
- the ability to **lyse** directly some bacteria and foreign cells
- **initiation of acute inflammation** by release of certain peptides (e.g. C3a and C5a) that act as chemotactic factors and induce vasodilatation with increased vascular permeability (anaphylatoxins). Additional roles include inducing smooth muscle contraction and causing mast cell degranulation
- solubilising and **removing immune complexes** from the circulation
- **prevention of cell entry** by bacteria and viruses.

- Heat labile PP
- Combine c Abs.
- Infl. response
- Both innate & adaptive immune responses.

Q46   Describe the structure and function of immunoglobulins

Immunoglobulins (Ig) are polypeptides that function as antibodies in the immune response. They are produced by **plasma cells**, a type of mature B lymphocyte. Plasma cells are of lymphoid lineage and are produced by and mature in the bone marrow. They comprise about 30% of circulating lymphocytes. As a rule, plasma cells require **both antigen and T lymphocytes** for activation but some antigens, such as bacterial lipopolysaccharide, are capable of activating them directly.

All immunoglobulins have the **same basic structure**. Each molecule consists of **two identical light chains** and **two identical heavy chains** linked by **disulphide bonds** (Figure 3). The antigen-binding segment (Fab) is important for antigen recognition, the crystallisable fragment (Fc) for immune cell binding. Papain divides Ig into Fab and Fc. The light chains may be either κ or λ, the heavy chains γ, α, μ, ε or δ. Heavy chain type determines immunoglobulin type, the different heavy chains corresponding to IgG, IgA, IgM, IgE and IgD respectively.

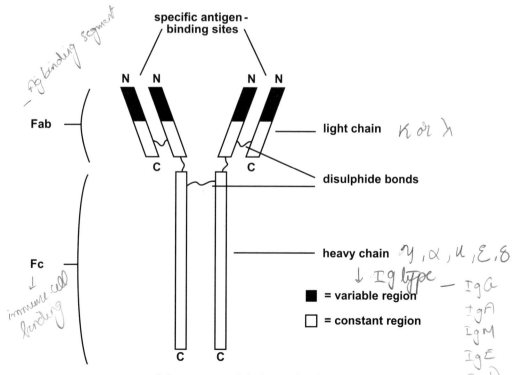

Figure 3   Basic structure of the immunoglobulin molecule. N = amino terminal; C = carboxyl terminal.

Table 9   Structure and function of immunoglobulins

	Structure	Comments	Complement activation
IgA	Dimeric	• Most abundant • Present in **exocrine secretions** such as tears and on mucosal surfaces such as the conjunctiva	Alternative pathway
IgD	Monomeric	• Precise functions unknown • Present as a surface receptor on lymphocytes • May be involved in B cell activation	
IgE	Monomeric	• Produced in larger amounts by **atopic** individuals • Bound mostly to mast cells • Antigen binding leads to **mast cell degranulation** • Has a role in **allergic responses** and the response to parasitic infections	Alternative pathway
IgG	Monomeric	• Most abundant (70–80%) Ig in the **blood and interstitial fluids** • Major Ig of the **secondary immune response** • Only Ig that **can cross the placenta** and is responsible for neonatal immunity • Has a role in **opsonising** foreign antigens	Classical pathway
IgM	Pentameric	• Mainly in the **intravascular** compartment • Principal Ig of the **primary immune response**	Strong complement activator via the classical pathway

Q47   Write short notes on histocompatibility antigens and list three examples of disease associations

Histocompatibility antigens

- These are part of the body's immune recognition system, and enable self antigens to be distinguished from non-self antigens.
- Important in transplant rejection.
- The most important group of histocompatibility antigens are the human leukocyte antigens (HLA), a series of cell surface glycoproteins coded for by the major histocompatibility complex (MHC) genes on the short arm of chromosome 6.
- There are two main MHC groups: classes I and II.

MHC class I molecules

- These are coded for by the HLA A, B and C loci, each of which can have multiple alleles.
- They are expressed on almost all cells except erythrocytes.
- Class I molecules comprise a heavy chain non-covalently linked to β_2-microglobulin.
- Each heavy chain has three domains: α_1, α_2 and α_3.
- The α_1 and α_2 domains lie distal to the cell membrane and consist of two α helices above a floor of β pleated sheet.
- This structure gives an overall appearance of a distinct groove.
- CD8-positive cytotoxic T cells recognise antigen in conjunction with MHC class I molecules.

MHC II molecules

- These are coded for by the DR, DP and DQ regions of the HLA complex.
- They are expressed principally on antigen-presenting cells such as macrophages and dendritic cells.
- CD4-positive T helper cells recognise antigen in conjunction with MHC class II molecules.
- Like MHC class I molecules, class II molecules also have a groove-like extracellular appearance.

Disease associations

These include:

- HLA-A29 and birdshot choroidoretinopathy (in 97% of cases)
- HLA-B27 and ankylosing spondylitis (90%)
- HLA-A11 and sympathetic ophthalmia
- HLA-B5 and Behçets disease.

Q48   Write short notes on the mechanism of allograft rejection

An **allograft** occurs when tissue is transferred between **two genetically different members of the same species**. Rejection is an immune process by which a graft is destroyed or rendered non-functional.

Five types of rejection are recognised, as shown in Table 10.

Table 10   Types of allograft rejection

	Onset	Mediators	Comments
Hyperacute	Within minutes	• Pre-formed humoral antibodies • Characterised by complement activation, polymorph infiltration and thrombus formation	• Infrequent with allografts, most common in xenografts • Serological cross-matching reduces the risk
Accelerated	Within 2–5 days	• Leads to memory B and T cell activation • Graft destruction is by cell-mediated immune mechanisms	• Only in those previously sensitised to donor antigen
Acute	Between 7 and 100 days	• Cell-mediated process • T cell stimulation results in a mononuclear macrophage response	• Occurs in hosts not previously sensitised to donor antigens
Chronic	More than 100 days	• Antibodies and complement are its main mediators • Inflammatory atheroma-like occlusion of graft blood vessels results in secondary donor organ ischaemia	
Acute on chronic		• T cell mediated	• Only occurs in the immunocompromised

Q49 Describe how antigen is presented to T lymphocytes

T lymphocytes are a part of the immune system involved in antigen recognition. T lymphocytes are (unable) to recognise antigen directly but require them to be 'presented' after being processed by antigen-presenting cells (APCs).

Antigen-presenting cells include the following:

- macrophages are large white blood cells that ingest antigens and other foreign substances which are then destroyed chemically or enzymatically after antigen presentation
- dendritic cells are the principal APCs of the primary immune response, although dendritic cells themselves do not actually mediate specific immune responses. Their major function is to obtain antigen in tissues before migrating to lymphoid organs where they activate T cells. Langerhans cells are dendritic cells specific to skin.

During antigen presentation the following steps occur:

- APCs engulf antigens by phagocytosis
- the antigen is broken down enzymatically into smaller fragments
- these smaller fragments are then transported to the surface of the APC bound with major histocompatibility complex (MHC) class II molecules
- in this processed form the antigen is recognised by T lymphocytes.

Q50   Discuss the local and systemic effects of neoplasia

Perhaps the best definition of neoplasia was in 1952 by the eminent British oncologist Sir Rupert Willis as 'an abnormal mass of tissue, the growth of which exceeds and is uncoordinated with that of normal tissues, and persists in the same excessive manner after cessation of the stimulus which evoked the change'.

Neoplasms may be benign or malignant, the key difference being that malignant neoplasms are capable of invasion and metastasis.

Local effects

The local effects of tumours are due to mechanical pressure displacing or compressing local structures and, in the case of malignant tumours, to tissue invasion and destruction. Local effects include:

- **mechanical pressure**, e.g. pancreatic cancer causing obstructive jaundice
- **destruction**, e.g. of bones, leading to pathological fractures
- **bleeding**, either acute or chronic – both occur with gastrointestinal tumours
- **secondary infection**, e.g. distal to a bronchial carcinoma.

Systemic

Tumours have both specific and non-specific systemic effects:

- **excess hormone production**, e.g. renal carcinoma producing erythropoietin
- **ectopic hormone production**, e.g. antidiuretic hormone (ADH) from bronchial tumours
- **cachexia** is more probably due to a cytokine effect than increased metabolic demands of the tumour
- **immune interaction**, e.g. non-metastatic lymphadenopathy
- **bone/joint/soft tissue**, e.g. clubbing or hypertrophic pulmonary osteoarthropathy in lung cancer
- **dermatological**, e.g. acanthosis nigricans in gastric cancer
- **neuropathies and myopathies** are common with carcinoma of the lung
- **vascular/haematological**, e.g. venous thrombosis and thrombophlebitis or anaemia
- **glomerular injury** can occur if immune complexes containing tumour antigen are deposited in the kidney.

Q51   Compare and contrast the innate and adaptive immune responses

Immunity means resistance to infection. Basic immune responses are divided into the innate or non-adaptive and the specific or adaptive responses. There are important similarities and differences between the two branches of the immune system, as outlined in Table 11.

Table 11   Innate and adaptive immune responses

Immune response	Innate	Adaptive
Principal components	• **Physical**, e.g. conjunctival epithelium, blink reflex • **Humoral**, e.g. tear lactoferrin, parts of the complement cascade • **Cellular**, e.g. macrophages and other phagocytic cells	Lymphocytes which focus and amplify parts of the innate immune system
Triggering molecules	Repetitive nucleotide repeats	Specific antigens
Recognition mechanism	Direct	Indirect
Clonal expansion of involved cells	No	Yes
Induces inflammation	Always	Sometimes
Onset	Hours	Days
Memory	No	Yes
Adaptability	No	Yes, able to respond to previously unseen antigens
Response to repeated exposure to the same antigen	Unchanged	Increased
Breadth of action	Narrow	Broad, although individual B and T cells are only able to respond to a limited number of antigens

Immune response	Innate	Adaptive
Specificity	Low	High
Site of action	Effective against extracellular antigens but very limited ability to combat intracellular infections	Greater capacity to respond to intracellular infections, particularly through T cells
Transferability between individuals	Not possible	Possible by transferring compatible lymphocytes or antibodies

Q52   Describe the histology of hypertensive vasculopathy

Hypertension **accelerates atherosclerosis**, the lesions having the same distribution and histological appearance as in non-hypertensive subjects.

Additionally, hypertension causes **thickening of the media** of muscular arteries and **collagen deposition** close to the internal elastic lamina. In contrast to the large arteries affected in atherosclerosis, **small and medium-sized vessels** are especially affected by hypertensive changes.

By causing increased transmural hydrostatic pressure gradients, hypertension also increases the normal protein flow into the vessel wall. High molecular weight proteins, such as fibrinogen, pass between endothelial cells resulting in extracellular protein deposition. In benign hypertension these deposits have a homogeneous appearance and are called **hyaline**. Hyaline changes are a common degenerative feature of many ageing arteries. In malignant hypertension **fibrinoid change** occurs: this is a combination of fibrin deposition and vessel wall necrosis.

Q53   Describe the structure and function of mitochondria

Mitochondria are egg-shaped intracellular organelles in which **oxidative phosphorylation** occurs. They comprise mostly protein but also lipid, deoxyribonucleic acid (DNA) and ribonucleic acid (RNA).

Their structure is visible under the electron microscope and consists of a **regular outer membrane surrounding an inner folded membrane**. The folds are known as cristae and are the site of oxidative phosphorylation and electron-transporting enzymes. Cristae are generally shelf-like but are tubular in steroid-secreting cells. The matrix lies central to the inner membrane and here the **maternally inherited double-stranded mitochondrial DNA** is found. In addition, the matrix contains enzymes of the **citric acid cycle** and of **fatty acid oxidation**.

By these processes mitochondria are involved in the **breakdown of glucose** to pyruvate, with concomitant production of **adenosine triphosphate** (ATP), the main energy currency of cells. Mitochondria are more numerous in cells such as heart muscle with high metabolic demands. The metabolic rate of individual mitochondria is related to the number of cristae they have.

New mitochondria are formed from old mitochondria when they grow and divide.

Mitochondrial DNA does not code for all mitochondrial proteins: some proteins are transported into mitochondria after synthesis on cytoplasmic ribosomes.

Q54   Write short notes on the bony anatomy of the orbit

Overview

- At the junction of the facial and cranial skeletons.
- **Seven bones** make up each orbit.
- Measure approximately 40 mm × 40 mm × 40 mm.
- Has the shape of a **square-based pyramid** with its base pointing anteriorly.
- The orbit is widest 1.5 cm behind the orbital rim and has a volume of 30 ml.
- The **medial walls are parallel**, the lateral walls each making an angle of 45° to this plane (i.e. 90° to each other).
- Major foramina entering the orbit include the superior and inferior orbital fissures and the optic canal.

Roof

- Relatively thin.
- Made up mostly by the **frontal bone** with the **lesser wing of the sphenoid** forming a smaller part posteriorly.
- Important superior relations are the frontal air sinuses and the anterior cranial fossa.
- Anterolaterally lies the fossa for the lacrimal gland, anteromedially the trochlea fossa, to which the pulley of superior oblique attaches.

Major foramina

- The optic canal runs through the lesser wing of the sphenoid bone at the apex of the orbit to connect with the middle cranial fossa.
- The superior orbital fissure lies between the lateral wall and roof of the orbit. It is comma shaped being bounded by the greater and lesser wings of the sphenoid bone and closed laterally by the frontal bone. It is the largest communication between the orbit and the middle cranial fossa.
- Between the floor and lateral wall is the inferior orbital fissure which connects the orbit to the infratemporal and pterygopalatine fossae.

Lateral wall

- **Thickest** orbital wall.
- Anterior one-third is made up by the **zygoma** and the posterior two-thirds by the **greater wing of the sphenoid**.
- Related anterolaterally to the temporal fossa and posterolaterally to the middle cranial fossa.
- No relationship with any air sinus.
- The frontozygomatic suture is one of the most common sites for dermoid cysts.
- Whitnall's tubercle, 11 mm below this suture, is the insertion of the lateral palpebral ligament, lateral check ligament, levator aponeurosis and suspensory ligament of the globe.

Floor

- 0.5–1 mm thick.
- Made up by the **maxillary**, **zygomatic** and **palatine** bones.
- Inferiorly lies the maxillary sinus.
- The floor is the orbital wall most frequently involved in blow-out fractures and subsequent entrapment of orbital fat often leads to restriction of upgaze.

Medial wall

- **Thinnest** of all (0.2–0.4 mm).
- Comprises, from anterior to posterior, the **frontal process of the maxilla**, **lacrimal**, **ethmoid** and **body of sphenoid** bones.
- Convex relative to the globe.
- The paper-thin lamina papricea separates the ethmoidal air cells from the orbit and infection can spread to the orbit following ethmoid sinusitis.

Q55   Write short notes on the blood supply to the anterior segment of the eye

Overview

The anterior segment of the eye includes the structures lying between the lens and cornea and includes the iris and ciliary body. Sometimes the conjunctiva and eyelids are also included in this definition.

Lens and cornea

- The lens and cornea are both avascular.
- The lens and inner corneal layers derive their nutrition from the aqueous humour.
- The corneal epithelium is nourished by nutrients in the tear film which diffuse from the limbal capillaries when the eye is open and from the palpebral capillaries when the eye is closed.

Iris and ciliary body

- The two long posterior ciliary arteries and the seven anterior ciliary arteries anastomose to form the major arterial circle which supplies the ciliary body.
- From this major circle radial arteries run into the iris, forming a minor circle at the iris collarette.
- Iris capillaries are non-fenestrated with endothelial tight junctions. In contrast, capillaries of the ciliary body are fenestrated and without endothelial tight junctions. The blood–aqueous barrier is maintained here by tight junctions between cells of the inner non-pigmented ciliary epithelium.
- Veins follow the arteries of the iris to form a corresponding minor circle. Radial veins do not form a corresponding major circle but rather converge and drain directly into the vortex veins.

Eyelids

- The eyelids are supplied by the lateral and medial palpebral arteries. The former is a branch of the lacrimal artery, itself a branch of the ophthalmic artery. The superior and inferior medial palpebral arteries arise from the ophthalmic artery just below the trochlea of superior oblique. After passing behind the lacrimal sac they enter the eyelids.

- Each artery divides into two branches forming two arches in each lid, a large marginal arch 3 mm from the free lid margin and a smaller peripheral arterial arch on the peripheral border of the tarsal plate.
- The eyelid blood vessels lie between orbicularis oculi and the tarsal plate.
- As well as anastomosing with the lateral palpebral arteries, the medial palpebral arteries have links with branches from the superficial temporal, transverse facial and infraorbital arteries.
- Thus the internal and external carotid artery systems anastomose in the eyelids.
- Eyelid veins are larger and more numerous than the arteries. Medially they drain into the angular and ophthalmic veins and laterally into the superficial temporal vein.

Conjunctiva

- The conjunctiva is supplied by the two palpebral arches of each eyelid and by the anterior ciliary arteries. The large marginal arch supplies the palpebral conjunctiva, and branches from the peripheral arch supply the fornices. Many vessels run from here under the bulbar conjunctiva to anastomose with the anterior conjunctival branches of the anterior ciliary arteries near the limbus.
- Again, conjunctival veins are larger and more numerous than the arteries. They reach the superior and inferior ophthalmic veins either directly or via the palpebral veins.

Q56 Outline the blood supply to the visual pathway

The visual pathway runs from the retina to the occipital cortex and its blood supply is from the internal carotid and the vertebro-basilar arterial systems. The two systems anastomose in the circle of Willis at the base of the brain.

Starting anteriorly, the blood supply to the visual pathway is described below:

- **retina**:
  - inner third by the central retinal artery
  - outer two-thirds by the long and short posterior ciliary arteries via the choroidal circulation
  - outer plexiform layer is at the junction between these two supplies
- **optic nerve**:
  - intraocular portion: short posterior ciliary arteries from the circle of Zinn
  - orbital portion: via the pial plexus from the ophthalmic artery. The central retinal artery also contributes
  - intracanalicular portion: via pial plexus from recurrent branches of the ophthalmic artery
  - intracranial portion: via pial plexus from the ophthalmic and superior hypophyseal arteries
- **optic chiasma**:
  - from the pial plexus, here supplied by branches of the internal carotid artery, superior hypophyseal artery and anterior and posterior communicating arteries
- **optic tract**:
  - from the pial plexus, here supplied by branches of the anterior choroidal and posterior communicating arteries
- **lateral geniculate nucleus**:
  - from the pial plexus, here supplied by the anterior choroidal branch of the middle cerebral artery, the thalamogeniculate branch of the posterior cerebral artery and the lateral choroidal artery
- **optic radiation**:
  - anteriorly by the anterior choroidal and middle cerebral arteries
  - posteriorly by the middle and posterior cerebral arteries
- **visual cortex**:
  - posterior and middle cerebral arteries, the latter anastomosing with the macular area.

The **internal carotid system is the main supply of the visual pathway from the retina to the optic radiation** and the **basilar artery from the optic radiation to the visual cortex**.

Q57   List the actions of the extraocular muscles and list the differences between extraocular muscles and other skeletal muscles

Table 12   Actions of the extraocular muscles

	*Primary action**	*Secondary action*
Medial rectus	Adduction	
Lateral rectus	Abduction	
Superior rectus	Elevation (maximal in abduction)	Adduction, intorsion
Inferior rectus	Depression (maximal in abduction)	Adduction, extorsion
Superior oblique	Intorsion	Elevation (maximal in adduction), abduction
Inferior oblique	Extorsion	Depression (maximal in adduction), abduction

*The primary actions described above are those of the muscle when it alone contracts in the primary position of gaze, i.e. the isolated agonist model.

Histologically, the extraocular muscles differ from other skeletal muscles in the following ways:

- the **muscle sheath**, or epimysium, of extraocular muscles is generally **very thin** in comparison to that of most skeletal muscles, except where it pierces the fasci bulbi
- the **fibres are not so tightly packed** but rather separated by unusually large amounts of connective tissue known as perimysium, which is rich in reticulin and elastic fibres
- extraocular muscle fibres are **rounded or oval in shape** with small fibres (5–15 μm) around their periphery and larger fibres (10–40 μm) in the centre
- extraocular muscles are the **most vascular muscles** in the body after the myocardium. Their most vascularised region is the orbital aspects.

Q58 Write short notes on the crystallins

- Crystallins make up the **majority of water-soluble protein** in the lens.
- **Classical crystallins** (alpha, beta and gamma crystallins) are present in all vertebrate lenses.
- **Alpha crystallins** represent one-third of lens proteins:
  - they are composed of **two subunits**, αA and αB
  - they are members of the **heat-shock protein family**
  - both subunits are **also expressed in other tissues in the body**
  - they have a **chaperone-like activity** whereby they bind to proteins that are beginning to unfold and prevent further unfolding and protein aggregation
  - since new protein synthesis is not possible in the nuclear lens fibres, it is thought that the chaperone activity of alpha crystallins is **important to maintain long-term lens transparency**.
- **Beta and gamma crystallins** were originally divided on the basis of different isoelectric points and aggregation properties. However, they have **homologous amino acid sequences** and **similar structures**:
  - beta crystallins are a complex group of oligomers
  - gamma crystallins are monomers which are expressed early in development and therefore are concentrated in the nucleus
  - **no specific biological functions** have been identified for beta and gamma crystallins, although some of them are **expressed outside the lens**
  - members of the superfamily have been identified in micro-organisms, where they are expressed during spore or cyst formation.
- **Taxon-specific crystallins** are expressed in large quantities in various phylogenetic groups (e.g. birds and reptiles). Most of these are **identical to known enzymes or related to major enzyme families**. Most taxon-specific crystallins are oxidoreductases.

Q59   Write short notes on carbohydrate metabolism in the lens

- Glucose enters the lens by both simple and facilitated diffusion.
- Most of the glucose is phosphorylated to **glucose-6-phosphate (G6P) by hexokinase**. This is the **rate-limiting step** for glycolysis in the lens:
  - G6P may enter the **glycolysis pathway** to form **pyruvate**, yielding two molecules of adenosine triphosphate (ATP) per molecule of glucose
  - G6P may enter the **hexose monophosphate shunt** (uses 5% of glucose) which **provides NADPH** [reduced nicotinamide adenine dinucleotide phosphate] necessary for continued production of **reduced glutathione**. The products of the hexose monophosphate shunt join the glycolysis pathway
  - pyruvate may be metabolised **anaerobically** to lactate or may enter the **Krebs cycle** and be metabolised aerobically
  - since the oxygen tension in the aqueous is low and since most fibres lack mitochondria, only about 3% of pyruvate enters the Krebs cycle to produce ATP. However, even this **low level of aerobic metabolism** provides 25% of the lens ATP
  - aerobic metabolism is more prominent in the lens epithelium and superficial lens fibres.
- Alternatively, glucose may be used by the **sorbitol pathway**:
  - under euglycaemic conditions about 5% of glucose is reduced to sorbitol by **aldose reductase**
  - sorbitol is then metabolised to fructose by polyol dehydrogenase. This enzyme has a low affinity; therefore in **hyperglycaemic** conditions, **large amounts of sorbitol** may accumulate which can cause **osmotic pressure**. This pathway is thought to be relevant to the formation of **diabetic cataracts**
  - similarly, in conditions of elevated galactose levels (i.e. **galactosaemia**), galactose may be reduced to **dulcitol** by aldose reductase. Dulcitol is not a substrate for polyol dehydrogenase and will accumulate, leading to **cataracts**.

Q60   List, with a brief explanation, the protective mechanisms against oxidative damage to the lens

Glutathione provides most of the protection against oxidative damage to the lens.

- Lowering the glutathione concentration in the lens experimentally produces cataracts.
- Its concentration in the lens is high, and its sulphydryl group is **readily oxidised**.
- Glutathione can also **reduce oxidised protein sulphydryl groups**.
- It is **synthesised in the lens epithelium and superficial lens fibres**. It is also transported into the lens from the aqueous. It **diffuses into the deeper fibres** from the superficial fibres. Conversely, oxidised glutathione (GSSG) must diffuse to the superficial lens fibres.
- Reduced glutathione is **regenerated by NADPH** [reduced nicotinamide adenine dinucleotide phosphate] and glutathione reductase.

Ascorbic acid also protects the lens from oxidative damage.

- Its concentration in the aqueous is **20 times** that in blood.
- Ascorbic acid may enter the lens through the glucose transporter. Ascorbic acid is **readily oxidised**, forming dehydroascorbate.
- Additionally, the high level of ascorbic acid in the aqueous (and the cornea) serves to **absorb ultraviolet B (UVB) radiation**.

Transferrin is present in high levels in the aqueous humour. Transferrin **binds iron** and prevents it from reacting with hydrogen peroxide to produce free radicals.

   Glutathione peroxidase and **catalase** are present in the lens epithelium and detoxify hydrogen peroxide.

Q61 Draw a dark adaptation curve and identify the component parts and their significance

Dark adaptation is the process by which the eye recovers its sensitivity to dim stimuli following exposure to bright light. To measure dark adaptation subjects are **fully light adapted** and then the change in **absolute visual threshold** is measured over time in the dark.

The curve is **biphasic**. The **initial rapid decrease is due to changes in cone sensitivity**. This slows and after 5–8 minutes a second rapid decrease in threshold occurs, followed by a slower decline. This **second phase is due to changes in rod sensitivity**. Complete dark adaptation takes about **40 minutes**.

Dark adaptation curves form the basis of the **duplicity theory** which states that above certain thresholds of illuminance the cone mechanism is principally responsible for mediating vision and below this cut-off the rod mechanism is more important. The transition range between the rod and cone mediated vision is called the **mesopic** range.

The significance of this is that in photopic conditions the high-energy light signal allows appreciation of colour, gives excellent central visual acuity and

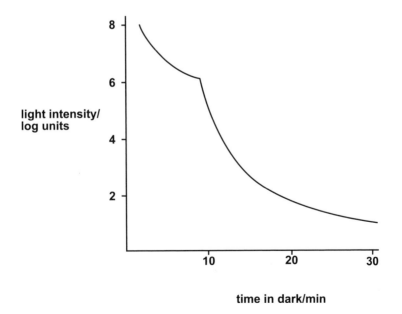

Figure 4 Dark adaptation curve: absolute visual threshold of a fully light-adapted subject after being placed in the dark (threshold against time).

relies on spatial summation with the signal being transmitted via the cone pathway. In rod-mediated scotopic vision visual acuity is poorer, colour vision absent and temporal summation of the light signal crucial. Thus in bright light the cone pathway predominates and in dim conditions the increased sensitivity of rods to light and their ability to use temporal summation mean they are most important.

Q62   Describe the mechanisms of visual adaptation

Overview

Visual adaptation is the process by which the visual system automatically adjusts visual sensitivity to changes in illumination so as to extract maximum contrast from the environment. Visual sensitivity can change by 12 log units and results in changes in temporal and spatial acuity and in spectral sensitivity.

Light adaptation

Light adaptation occurs when a dark-adapted person moves into the light. Light adaptation is rapid and gets faster when the light is brighter. Three processes are involved:

- the **pupil constricts** from a maximum of 9 mm to a minimum of 1 mm, reducing light entry by about 1.3 log unit. This takes less than 1 second
- **retinal neuronal light sensitivity** is altered within milliseconds by neural factors and can change by about 3 log units. It is thought that horizontal cells feed back on cones to reduce their light sensitivity. This effect is most pronounced with large diffuse stimuli
- **photochemical changes** lead to the greatest change in visual sensitivity (8 log units) but take seconds to minutes to occur. Light exposure leads to photopigment bleaching: the molecular basis of this process is thought to involve changes in intracellular calcium levels. At normal levels of ambient lighting approximately 5% of rhodopsin is bleached.

The light-adapted eye is maximally sensitive to light of wavelength 555 nm.

Dark adaptation

Dark adaptation is slower than light adaptation. Changes in pupil size and retinal neural activity occur as described above, just in reverse. Unbleaching of photopigments is slower than bleaching and leads to a biphasic increase in light sensitivity that occurs due to the different rates of recovery of rods and cones. There is an initial rapid increase in sensitivity due to changes in cone sensitivity. After about 8 minutes a second rapid increase in sensitivity occurs due to changes in rod sensitivity. It takes 30 minutes for rhodopsin to fully regenerate. The dark-adapted eye is maximally sensitive to light of wavelength 505 nm and at absolute threshold can detect 4–10 quanta absorbed/degree/100 ms.

Q63   What is known of the function of retinal pigment epithelial cells?

The retinal pigment epithelium (RPE) is a monolayer of cuboidal/columnar epithelium lying between the photoreceptor layer of the retina and Bruch's membrane of the choroid. RPE cells are hexagonal on tangential section.

Functions of the RPE cells include:

- biochemical:
  - uptake, transport, storage, metabolism and isomerisation of vitamin A
  - recognition, ingestion and phagocytosis of shed photoreceptor outer segment tips
  - detoxification of drugs
  - free radical scavenging
  - synthesis of melanin and extracellular matrices
- physiological:
  - homeostasis of the photoreceptor environment
  - selective transport of water and metabolites to and from the retina
  - immunoregulation
- physical and optical:
  - promotion of retinal adherence
  - maintenance of the outer blood–retinal barrier
  - absorption of stray light to reduce scatter.

Q64 Write short notes on the electrophysiological investigations of the visual pathway

Electro-oculogram (EOG)

Principle function

Records corneo-retinal potential.

Technique

Electrodes are placed at the medial and lateral canthi. The subject performs 30° lateral eye movements at regular intervals during a period of dark adaptation, approximately 20 minutes, followed by a shorter period of light adaptation.

Interpretation

The amplitude of the signal reaches a minimum in the dark – the dark trough – and rises to a maximum in the light – the light peak. The critical value is the **Arden ratio** (light peak : dark trough), which is normally greater than 80%.

Change in disease

Changes in the EOG usually parallel changes seen in the electroretinogram (ERG), a notable exception being Best's vitelliform macular dystrophy when the EOG is abnormal but the ERG normal. The relationship of the EOG to physiological functions of the retinal pigment epithelium (RPE) is unclear as it does not correlate with pigmentary changes or visual function.

Electroretinogram (ERG)

Principle function

Records the electrical mass response of the retina to light stimulation.

Technique

Use of corneal electrodes (e.g. contact lens electrode) to measure the response of the light- or dark-adapted retina to single or repetitive flashes. Five types of ERG are usually performed:

1   maximal combined response to a single flash of light
2   **scotopic** ERG (in which dim light below cone threshold is used to isolate rod response)
3   **photopic** (with a bright background to saturate rods, giving a cone-only response)
4   56 Hz **flicker** (only cones can respond to frequencies higher than 20 Hz)
5   **oscillatory** (isolated by filtering out slower components of the ERG; result from interactions in the inner nuclear and plexiform layers).

Interpretation

The **a wave** is a corneal negative deflection thought to be produced by the photoreceptors. It is followed by the corneal positive **b wave** generated by the Muller cells, which act as a 'sink' for potassium ions released by depolarising bipolar cells. Changes in the amplitude of these waves reflect absence or abnormality of populations of photoreceptors (a wave) or the inner retina (b wave). Additionally, the subtype of photoreceptor population may be identified (rods or cones or both).

Pattern ERG (pERG)

The principle and technique are as for the ERG except that the stimulus presented is a reversing alternating pattern of black and white checks.

The pERG has two main components, P_{50} and N_{95}, the letter referring to the positive or negative polarity of the response and the numerical subscript to the time to peak response (ms). P_{50} is reduced by inner retina and ganglion cell damage, N_{95} by optic nerve disease.

The pERG is less dominated by the fovea than visually evoked potentials because the amplitude of the response varies with cell density per unit area.

Visually evoked potentials (VEP)

Principle function

The VEP measures the cortical response to light stimulation.

Technique

Cortical electrodes are applied. The usual stimulus is a reversing chequerboard or, less commonly, a single bright flash.

Interpretation

Latency of the response is the most useful clinical parameter. It is increased in a variety of disorders, including optic nerve demyelination, compressive lesions and ischaemic lesions. VEP is delayed in macular lesions.

Q65   Describe the absorption of ultraviolet, visible and infrared light by the eye and discuss their harmful effects

Overview

- Visible light has wavelengths of 400–760 nm.
- Infrared (IR) light has longer wavelengths (760–10^5 nm), ultraviolet (UV) shorter (200–400 nm).
- Energy of light is proportional to the reciprocal of its wavelength: this makes UV light more harmful than IR.

Light absorption

- Infrared:
  - the cornea absorbs nearly all IR light of wavelength greater than 1400 nm
  - IR light is also absorbed by pigmented structures such as the iris, trabecular meshwork and choroid.
- Visible:
  - the eye has evolved to ensure the minimum of visible light is absorbed by the optical media and the maximum of light reaches the retinal photoreceptors. However, absorption of stray light by pigmented structures, in particular the choroid, prevents reflection and scatter which would otherwise reduce image quality
  - xanthophyll macular pigments reduce glare by absorbing short-wavelength blue light.
- Ultraviolet:
  - the cornea absorbs 45% of light of less than 280 nm wavelength but only 12% of light with wavelengths 320–420 nm
  - longer wavelength UV light is absorbed by the yellow pigments of the lens. The amount of these yellow pigments increases with age and more blue and UV light reaches the retinae of children than of adults.

Light-related ocular injury

- Skin:
  - acutely UV light causes sunburn; long-term excess exposure can cause basal and squamous cell carcinomas and malignant melanomas by causing deoxyribonucleic acied (DNA) mutations.
- Cornea and conjunctiva:
  - the cornea is most sensitive to UV light of wavelength 270 nm. This causes a transient superficial punctate keratitis 8–12 hours after exposure ('arc eye'). Chronic UV exposure is implicated in the development of pterygia and pingueculae.
- Lens:
  - cataracts, especially anterior cortical, are related to extended UV exposure.
- Retina:
  - photoreceptors are particularly vulnerable to free radical mediated damage. Free radical production is increased by exposure to light, in particular UV light
  - IR radiation causes macular damage in sungazers
  - light-related injury has been suggested as a cause of age-related macular degeneration.

Q66 Describe the retinotopic organisation of the visual pathway. Use an image in the left superior visual field as an example

Retina

- An image in the left superior visual field projects onto the inferonasal retina of the left eye and the inferotemporal retina of the right eye.
- Photoreceptors synapse with bipolar cells which in turn synapse with ganglion cells.

Optic nerve

- Axons of ganglion cells form the optic nerve and proceed posteriorly to the optic chiasma.
- In the optic nerve peripheral retinal fibres are arranged exactly as they are in the retina: temporal fibres lie laterally, nasal fibres medially.
- At the origin of the optic nerve macular fibres form a wedge laterally. Macular fibres come to lie in the centre of the nerve by the time it approaches the optic chiasma.

Optic chiasma

- At the optic chiasma fibres from the nasal retina decussate but those from the temporal retina do not.
- Crossed and uncrossed fibres are intermingled within the posterior chiasma.
- In this example, fibres from the left inferonasal retina decussate to lie on the same side as those from the right inferotemporal retina which do not decussate.

Optic tract

- The lateral root of the optic tract is concerned with conscious visual function and terminates in the lateral geniculate nucleus (LGN) of the thalamus.

- In the optic tract:
  - fibres corresponding to the inferior retina lie laterally
  - fibres from the upper retina are positioned medially
  - macular fibres lie posterolaterally.
- The lateral root of the optic tract rotates 90° inwards before reaching the LGN.

Lateral geniculate nucleus

- Fibres from the ipsilateral eye project to layers 2, 3 and 5 of the LGN and fibres from the contralateral eye project to layers 1, 4 and 6.
- The LGN is retinotopically mapped:
  - fibres from the superior retina project to its medial aspect
  - inferior retinal fibres project laterally
  - the macula projects posteriorly and the peripheral retina anteriorly.
- In the above example the image is projected to the right LGN: fibres from the inferonasal left retina project to its lateral aspect in layers 1, 4 and 6 and fibres from the inferotemporal right retina project to the lateral aspect of layers 2, 3 and 5.

Optic radiation

- The nerve fibres of cells whose bodies lie in the LGN form the optic radiation, which runs to the ipsilateral visual cortex in Brodman area 17 in the occipital lobe.
- The retinotopic organisation of the LGN is maintained in the optic radiation:
  - fibres representing superior retina lie posteriorly
  - the anterior fibres correspond to inferior retina
  - macular fibres lie medially.

Primary visual cortex

- Fibres of the optic radiation terminate in layer 4 of the primary visual cortex.
- The retinotopic mapping of the visual cortex is as follows:
  - the inferior hemiretina projects to the inferior lip of the calcarine sulcus
  - the superior retina is represented on the superior lip of the calcarine sulcus
  - the macula projects to the posterior 30% of both lips.
- An image in the left superior visual field projects to the inferior lip of the calcarine sulcus in the right occipital lobe.

Q67   Write short notes on the classification of visual acuity

To measure visual acuity is to measure the spatial limits of visual discrimination and involves the determination of thresholds. There are several different ways of classifying visual acuity:

- **minimum visible** ('is that object visible or not?'):
  - requires detection of a visible stimulus against a uniform background
  - can be achieved at visual angles of 1 second of arc or less
  - changes in object size below 1 minute of arc visual angle are perceived as variation in contrast and not size
- **minimum resolvable** ('is that one object or two?'):
  - a measure of the ability to distinguish two stimuli as being separate
  - relies on detection of contrast differences between retinal 'detecting units'
  - greatest at the fovea and least in the periphery
  - at threshold it corresponds to between 30 seconds and 1 minute of visual angle
- **minimum discriminate** (Vernier acuity or hyperacuity):
  - is the determination of the relative locations of two or more visible points
  - threshold of hyperacuity is 3–12 seconds of visual arc
  - possible despite a minimum cone separation at the fovea of 1 minute of arc due to cortical processing
- **stereoacuity**:
  - stereoacuity is the smallest binocular disparity that can be reliably detected
  - threshold for stereoacuity is 3–12 seconds of arc, similar to hyperacuity.

Q68   Discuss the cortical contribution to visual function

The cortex makes important contributions to both visual perception and to the control of eye movements.

Eye movements

Although the oculomotor nuclei and final common pathways for horizontal and vertical eye movements are subcortical, cortical centres have an important role in the control of eye movements:

- horizontal saccades originate in the contralateral frontal eye fields of the frontal cortex and are independent of visual stimuli
- pursuit movements originate from the occipitoparietal cortex, where stimulation leads to conjugate eye movement towards the other side
- the temporal cortex, as a centre for relay for motion information, is important in saccadic eye movements to moving objects. It is also involved in the initial detection of objects prior to voluntary fixation.

Visual perception

The primary visual cortex (V_1) is situated on the lips of the calcarine sulcus on the medial aspect of the occipital lobe. It is the site of termination of neurones originating in the lateral geniculate and is the most important part of the visual processing system. Without it visual perception does not occur. There are cells in the visual cortex specialised for colour, object length and orientation detection. Contrast detection is enhanced by the existence of cells with 'centre–surround' type visual fields.

Several supplemental areas of visual cortex exist, important for detailed visual analysis and each with its own sub-specialisation:

- V_2 is important for colour analysis
- V_5 is particularly sensitive to motion and object orientation but has no sensitivity to colour.

The sensory speech area of Wernicke, usually found in the left dominant hemisphere, mainly on the superior temporal gyrus, permits the understanding of written and spoken language and enables a person to read a sentence, understand it and say it out loud.

Other cortical areas play roles in visual memory and object identification.

Q69   Write short notes on the normal visual field and how it can be measured

Overview

- The monocular visual field is the proportion of external space visible to a single stationary eye from the primary position of gaze and extends approximately 50° superiorly, 60° nasally, 70° inferiorly and 90° temporally.
- There is a physiological blind spot about 10–20° temporal to the centre of the visual field which corresponds to the area of the optic nerve head where photoreceptors are absent.
- Visual acuity is greatest near the centre of the visual field and declines towards the periphery.
- Scotomas are absolute or relative visual field defects. A scotoma is said to be positive if the patient is aware of it and negative if they are not.
- Characteristic field losses occur in particular pathological conditions such as arcuate field losses in glaucoma or enlarged blind spots in optic neuritis.

Confounding factors

Miosis, lens opacities, ptosis and refractive errors all lead to potential sources of error during visual field testing.

Measurement variables

Larger stimuli are more readily seen than smaller stimuli. The lower spatial acuity of the peripheral retina means that the visual field reduces in size when measured with smaller stimulus sizes.

The colour of the stimulus and its background may affect stimulus perception.

Measurement techniques

Perimetric visual field testing involves the use of a partial sphere, such as the Ganz field screen, in which the test object remains a constant distance from the eye. For compimetry, a flat (Bjerrum) screen is used and object distance increases peripherally.

During kinetic testing a target of fixed size and luminance is moved towards the centre of the visual field until it is seen. Static testing involves a fixed target of a particular size being shown for the same period of time at different luminances until seen. Static testing is slower than kinetic testing but it is much better suited to quantitative visual field testing.

Clinical measurement of the visual field

Confrontation field testing is rapid and requires no specialised equipment, making it an excellent screening test for gross field defects.

The Goldmann perimeter is a manually operated kinetic field analyser. It requires a skilled operator and is slow but is the gold-standard measure of the visual field.

The Humphrey perimeter is a widely used automated field analyser which tests by static perimetry and gives a computerised printout of its findings and their reliability.

Q70   Write short notes on the principles of intraocular pressure measurement

- Measurements of intraocular pressure (IOP) are either **direct** or **indirect**.
- **Direct measurement** of IOP involves insertion of a pressure transducer into the anterior chamber (manometry). This is **not used clinically**.
- **Indirect measurement** is **used clinically**:
  - in **applanation tonometry**, the **cornea is flattened** and IOP is determined by measuring the applanating force and the area flattened $(P = F/A)$ The **Goldmann tonometer** measures the **force required to flatten an area of cornea 3.06 mm in diameter**. This is the diameter at which the resistance of an average thickness cornea is counterbalanced by the capillary forces of the tear film. Fluorescein in the tear film is used to allow precise estimation of the area of flattening. The Goldmann applanation tonometer is used with a slitlamp and is the **most accurate** method currently available. The Perkins tonometer is a portable tonometer which uses applanation to measure the IOP in the supine or erect patient. Portable electronic applanation devices employ a similar principle but flatten a smaller area of cornea
  - **non-contact tonometers** (air-puff tonometers) determine the IOP by measuring **the time needed for a given force of air to flatten a known area of cornea**
  - **indentation tonometry** is based on the calculation of IOP from **the degree of corneal deformation produced by a given force.** Indentation is measured by the degree of excursion of the instrument's plunger, and converted to IOP values by means of a calibrated scale on the instrument or from a conversion table. The **Schiotz tonometer** is the most commonly used such instrument.

Q71   Discuss the mechanisms of aqueous secretion and their modification by drugs

- Most aqueous humour is produced by the **ciliary epithelium**:
  - at approximately 2 μl/minute
  - 65–85% by active secretion
  - 5–15% by ultrafiltration
  - about 10% by osmosis
  - about 8% by the corneal endothelial pump.
- The ciliary epithelium is a bilayer of apically opposed cells:
  - the inner layer is non-pigmented and the outer layer pigmented
  - cells of the inner layer of ciliary epithelium are linked by tight junctions
  - the inner layer has the major role in aqueous production but aqueous production does continue after its selective ablation.
- **Active secretion** is thought to be responsible for most of aqueous secretion for several reasons:
  - the blood–aqueous barrier formed by tight junctions between the inner non-pigmented ciliary epithelium acts as a relative barrier to aqueous production
  - aqueous and plasma have significant chemical differences in composition
  - ouabain, which inhibits the Na–K ATPase active pump, reduces aqueous production by 70%.
- The mechanism of active aqueous secretion involves:
  - passive diffusion of Na and Cl across the ciliary epithelium
  - this is driven by concentration gradients established by the Na–K ATPase pump and is dependent on the action of **carbonic anhydrase type 2**
  - aqueous production is under **adrenergic control**
  - the predominant adrenoreceptors are β_2 and their stimulation leads to reduced aqueous production.
- Drugs which modify active aqueous secretion can act at any point in this process:
  - reduction in aqueous production leads to a fall in intraocular pressure
  - carbonic anhydrase inhibitors such as acetazolamide reduce aqueous production by up to 50%
  - β-blockers like timolol reduce aqueous secretion as do α_2-agonists like apraclonidine.
- Ultrafiltration and osmosis are passive processes which have less of a role than active secretion in aqueous production:
  - no clinical agents in current use to reduce intraocular pressure act in this way

– drugs which reduce systemic blood pressure or increase plasma osmolality theoretically reduce aqueous production by this route but in practice such drugs reduce intraocular pressure by increasing aqueous outflow.

Q72   Write short notes on the supranuclear control of eye movements

Overview

- The four principal supranuclear subsystems involved in control of eye movements are the saccadic, pursuit, vergence and vestibular systems.
- The description here is an oversimplification and the role of the cerebellum in visual coordination and of cortical regions such as the secondary visual cortex in other aspects of the process will not be discussed.

Saccadic

- Saccadic eye movements are under both voluntary and involuntary control.
- Saccades are the fastest of eye movements and have a velocity of up to $400°$ per second.
- Stimulus is target displacement and results in a burst of stimulation to the appropriate agonist muscle with total inhibition of its antagonist.
- Horizontal saccades are controlled by the **frontal eye fields** (FEF) in area 8 of the frontal cortex from where impulses pass to the **parapontine reticular formation** (PPRF), the start of the final common pathway of horizontal eye movements, and onto the various oculomotor nuclei.
- The **vestibular nuclei** are involved in the initiation of vertical saccades.
- The vertical gaze centre is less well understood but is thought to lie in the **rostral interstitial nucleus** of the medial longitudinal fasciculus (MLF) in the midbrain.
- The MLF links the nuclei of the third, fourth, sixth and eighth cranial nerves.

Pursuit

- Pursuit eye movements occur in response to movement of a fixated target.
- Pursuit movements have a latency of 125 ms and a velocity of up to $100°$ per second.
- They are smooth in nature and under control of systems capable of continuous modification.
- Pursuit movements are under control of the **ipsilateral occipitoparietal cortex**.

Vergence

- In convergence movements the eyes move towards each other; in divergence movements they move apart.
- Convergence usually occurs as part of the accommodation reflex.
- The trigger for vergence movements is target displacement or motion along the axis parallel to the direction of gaze.

Vestibular

- Triggered by head movements, vestibular eye movements result in a shift in gaze away from the direction of movement.
- The inner ear detects both rotational and linear acceleration and transmits this information to the vestibular nuclei of the midbrain via the vestibulocochlear nerve.
- From this nucleus signals pass to the appropriate oculomotor nuclei through the MLF.
- The vestibulocochlear reflex tests the integrity of the vestibular eye movement control system.

Clinical notes

- Intranuclear ophthalmoplegia (INO) is the most common disorder of supranuclear control of eye movements.
- In INO there is a lesion in the part of the MLF linking the third and sixth cranial nerve nuclei on contralateral sides, resulting in a failure of adduction on the affected side with nystagmus in the contralateral adducting eye.
- Multiple sclerosis and strokes are the most common causes of unilateral intranuclear ophthalmoplegia.

Q73   Describe the mechanism of colour perception

Historical perspective

During the nineteenth century there were two main rival theories of colour vision.

Young, Helmholz and Maxwell's **trichromatic theory** proposed that there are three distinct classes of cones, each sensitive to light of slightly different wavelengths, and that perceived colour depends on the relative stimulation of each class of cone.

- The trichromatic theory is based on the observation that, in those with normal colour vision, any colour can be matched using different proportions of three monochromatic lights.
- Direct confirmatory evidence of the existence of three different wavelength-sensitive cone subclasses has been obtained by microspectrophotometry. Cones can be subdivided into those with short-, medium- and long-wavelength peak sensitivities which correspond to 'blue', 'green' and 'red' cones respectively.

Opposing the trichromatic theory, Hering advanced the **opponent theory** based on empiric observations that certain colour pairings are mutually exclusive and do not yield composite visual sensations. For example, mixing of red and green light yields yellow and mixing of yellow and blue light yields white light.

Current thinking

It has now been established that both the trichromatic and opponent theories are correct:

- at the photoreceptor level colour vision is trichromatic
- from ganglion cells and beyond there are two main classes of opponent cells:
  - opponent cells have simple receptive fields: their firing is stimulated by light of one colour and inhibited by light of another
  - double opponent cells have a more complicated 'centre–surround' visual field: the central part of their visual field is stimulated by one

colour and inhibited by another colour and the surrounding area has the opposite properties. Such cells are well suited to identifying object borders and contrast.

Although perceived colour is fundamentally influenced by the wavelength of light reflected from an object, it is not determined by the wavelength of that light. **Colour constancy** is the phenomenon whereby the perceived colour of an object appears constant despite wide variations in the wavelength of illuminating light. The mechanism of colour constancy is poorly understood but involves higher cerebral centres and contrast with surrounding objects.

Q74   Draw a cross-section of the upper eyelid. Label all important structures and write short notes on each

The eyelids have a six-layered structure. From superficial to deep these layers are:

- **skin**:
  - thinnest on the body
  - insertion of some of the fibres of levator palpebrae superioris causes the upper lid skin crease
- **subcutaneous tissue**:
  - there is no subcutaneous fat
  - extracellular fluid or blood can accumulate in this layer
- **orbicularis oculi**:
  - innervated by the facial nerve
  - palpebral fibres are responsible for reflex blinking
- **loose areolar tissue**:
  - the neurovascular bundle runs here
- **tarsal plate**:
  - 10 mm in height
  - thickening of the orbital septum forming the fibrous framework of the eyelid

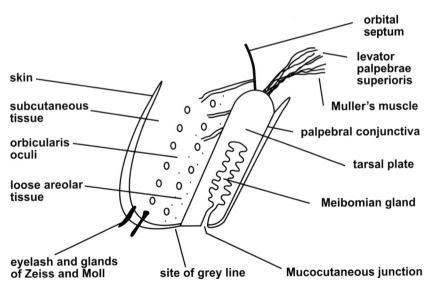

Figure 5   Cross-section through the upper eyelid.

- each upper lid contains the 35 or so Meibomian glands. These modified sebaceous glands secrete the lipid outer layer of the tear film. Meibomian gland orifices are at the mucocutaneous junction lying behind the eyelashes
- levator palpebrae superioris inserts into the tarsal plate. It is innervated by the superior division of the oculomotor nerve and acts to elevate the upper lid
- Muller's muscle also inserts into the tarsal plate: it originates from the posterior aspect of levator palpebrae superioris. Muller's muscle is innervated by the sympathetic nervous system and elevates the upper lid by about 2 mm
- **palpebral conjunctiva**:
  - firmly adherent to the tarsal plate and in continuity with the forniceal conjunctiva.

The grey line marks a relatively avascular plane along which the eyelid can be split into an anterior layer of skin, subcutaneous tissue and orbicularis oculi muscle and posterior lamella of tarsal plate and conjunctiva.

Q75   Describe the structure and function of the conjunctiva

The conjunctiva is a transparent mucous membrane lining the ocular surface, linking the globe and eyelids. It is derived from ectoderm and has three parts:

- **bulbar**: the bulbar conjunctiva lies loosely over the sclera and merges with the corneal epithelium about 1 mm anterior to the corneoscleral limbus and fuses with Tenon's capsule approximately 3 mm posterior to the limbus
- **palpebral**: this is firmly adherent to the tarsal plates
- **forniceal**: the tarsal conjunctiva forms outpouchings between the bulbar and palpebral conjunctivae. The superior fornix extends about 10 mm from the limbus, inferior 8 mm and lateral 14 mm (i.e. behind the equator). There is no medial fornix.

Histologically, conjunctival tissue comprises a **stratified non-keratinised epithelium** containing connective tissue, blood vessels, plasma cells, accessory lacrimal glands and lymphoid follicles. Most of the conjunctival epithelial cells are columnar but near the corneal limbus and mucocutaneous junction they become squamous. Goblet cells are most numerous on the inferonasal bulbar conjunctiva.

Innervation is principally by the **ophthalmic division of the trigeminal nerve**, although the maxillary division contributes inferonasally.

Functions of the conjunctiva include:

- **tear production** by the goblet cells and accessory lacrimal tissues
- **protection** both by being a physical barrier to infection and also through the ability of epithelial cells to phagocytose foreign materials and bacteria
- the vascular and lymphoid channels present in the conjunctiva form the afferent and efferent arms of the humoral and cellular **immune responses**. The conjunctiva is also part of the mucosa-associated lymphoid tissue (MALT) and produces secretory immunoglobulin A (IgA).

Q76   Draw a diagram of the anterior chamber drainage angle and write short notes on the anatomy of the structure

Ninety percent of aqueous drains via the anterior chamber drainage angle. Total internal reflection of light from the angle on the cornea prevents angle structures from being seen directly. This can be overcome if a material with a greater refractive index than the cornea, such as a gonioscopy lens, is placed on its anterior surface.

From anterior to posterior, the following structures may be seen on gonioscopy:

- **Schwalbe's line**, the posterior termination of Descemet's membrane, appears as an opaque line and lies anterior to the commencement of the trabecular meshwork
- the **corneal wedge** coincides with Schwalbe's line. It can be identified on gonioscopy as the point where the reflections of a narrow slitlamp beam from the internal and external corneal surfaces meet
- the **trabecular meshwork**, which contains Schlemm's canal and is attached to the scleral spur. In certain pathological conditions the trabeculum becomes hyperpigmented
- the **canal of Schlemm** can be seen in some eyes without trabecular pigmentation as a slightly darker line deep to the posterior trabeculum. Schlemm's canal is lined by endothelium and aqueous passes into it in vacuoles formed from the endothelium of the trabecular meshwork. It is not in direct communication with the aqueous

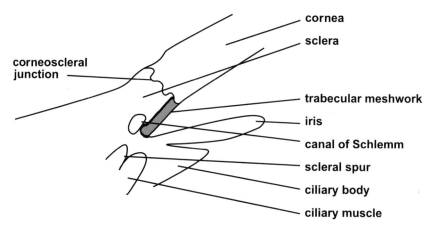

Figure 6   The drainage angle of the anterior chamber.

- the **scleral spur** is one of the most consistent angle landmarks between individuals. It is seen as a shiny white band of sclera running between the trabecular meshwork and ciliary body. The longitudinal muscle fibres of the ciliary muscle insert into the scleral spur
- the anterior face of the **ciliary body** is marked by a pigmented band. Its width depends on the position of iris insertion
- **iris processes** can be seen in about one-third of eyes. Iris processes are small insertions of the anterior iris surface which insert at the level of the scleral spur. They are less common with increasing age
- normal **blood vessels** run in a radial direction at the base of the angle recess. Pathological blood vessels may run in any direction.

Q77   Describe the structure and function of the ciliary body

Overview

The ciliary body is the middle part of the uveal tract and is continuous anteriorly with the periphery of the iris and posteriorly with the choroid. The ciliary body forms a ring that runs around the inside of the anterior sclera, measuring about 6 mm wide (6.5 mm temporally, 5.5 mm nasally) and extending forward to the scleral spur and backward to the ora serrata. The surface landmark of the anterior aspect of the ciliary body is the point 1.5 mm posterior to the corneal limbus.

Gross anatomy

The ciliary body is triangular in cross-section with its small base facing the anterior chamber. The anterior portion is ridged and called the pars plicata; the posterior portion is flat and known as the pars plana. The pars plicata gives rise to the ciliary processes to which the zonules of the lens attach and it surrounds the periphery of the iris. The pars plana has a scalloped posterior border that fits into the scalloped edge of the retina at the ora serrata.

Microscopic anatomy

The ciliary body has three layers.

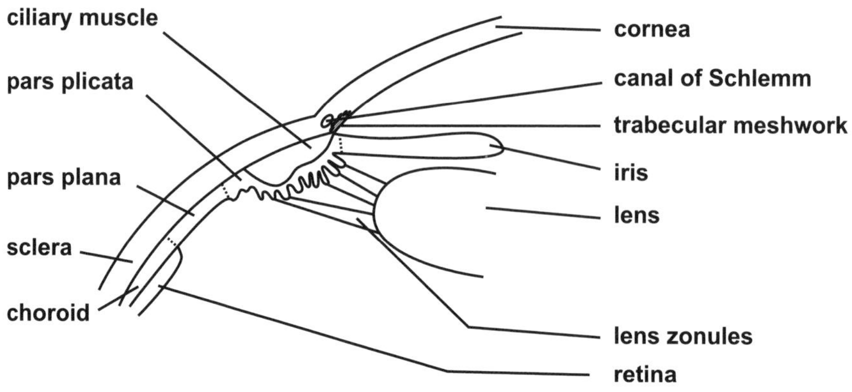

Figure 7   Gross anatomy of the ciliary body.

- The ciliary epithelium is a bilayer of cuboidal cells, arranged apex to apex, covering the inner surface of the ciliary body. Embryologically, the bilayer represents the two layers of the optic cup. The inner layer is non-pigmented and the outer layer pigmented. Tight junctions between cells of the inner layer form an important part of the blood–aqueous barrier.
- The ciliary stroma consists of bundles of loose connective tissue rich in blood vessels and melanocytes in which the ciliary muscle is embedded. The connective tissue extends into the core of the ciliary processes. Blood vessels present include the ciliary arteries, veins and capillaries. A major arterial circle lies at the iris root. The endothelium of the capillaries close to the ciliary epithelium is fenestrated.
- The ciliary muscle forms the bulk of the substance of the ciliary body. It is a smooth muscle. Most fibres attach to the scleral spur and fall into three groups: longitudinal (passing into the choroidal stroma), circular (the most interior forming a sphincter) and radial (linking the other two layers). The muscle is innervated by postganglionic parasympathetic fibres via the short ciliary nerves.

Functions

- The ciliary epithelium, in particular its inner layer, is responsible for aqueous secretion.
- The ciliary body probably secretes glycosaminoglycan into the vitreous from its posterior surface.
- Contraction of the ciliary muscle causes accommodation by relaxing the tension in the zonules, allowing the lens to assume a more convex shape and so increasing the refractive power of the eye.

Q78   Describe the lacrimal gland. Include a short note on its development

The lacrimal gland:

- is situated anterolaterally in the **roof of the orbit**
- measures $5 \times 12 \times 20$ mm
- has **two parts**: a larger orbital part in the lacrimal fossa of the orbital roof and a smaller palpebral part lying below the aponeurosis of levator palpebrae superioris:
  - the palpebral part is one-third the size of the orbital part
  - the two parts of the gland are continuous with one another and do not lie within a definitive capsule
- secretes the aqueous component of **tears**, with those produced by the orbital part passing through the palpebral part before release via 9–12 small ducts into the conjunctival sac
- removal of the palpebral part leads to the gland becoming non-secreting
- receives **parasympathetic secretomotor** supply:
  - derived from the superior salivatory nucleus of the seventh cranial nerve
  - reaches the pterygopalatine ganglion through the nervus intermedius and its greater petrosal branch
  - post-ganglionic fibres run in the zygomaticotemporal and then lacrimal nerves
- also receives sympathetic and sensory innervation
- arterial supply is via the lacrimal artery, from the ophthalmic artery
- venous drainage is into the ophthalmic vein
- lymphatic drainage joins that of the conjunctiva and passes into the superficial parotid nodes
- **lobulated tubuloacinar structure**:
  - smaller ducts are lined by a monolayer of low columnar or cuboidal epithelium, larger ducts by a bilayer
  - both parts have myoepithelial cells at their periphery
  - secretory cells have **basally located nuclei**
  - most secretory cells are of the serous type but some mucus-producing cells are also present
- forms from a series of **ectodermal** buds that grow superolaterally from the superior fornix of the conjunctiva into the underlying mesenchyme. Development of levator palpebrae superioris muscle divides the gland into lacrimal and orbital parts.

Q79   Discuss the anatomy of the cerebellum, including its blood supply and neuronal connections

Overview

- The cerebellum is situated in the posterior cranial fossa and comprises two lateral hemispheres separated by the midline vermis.
- It is linked to the brainstem by three pairs of cerebellar peduncles.
- The most anterior and caudal part of the lateral lobe is the flocculus, attached to a nodule in the midline. Together they form the flocculo-nodular lobe, an important part of the vestibular system and involved in the maintenance of balance.
- The bulge of the lateral lobe which projects inferiorly posterolateral to the medulla is the tonsil and in cases of raised intracranial pressure the tonsils can herniate through the foramen magnum and compress the medulla oblongata ('coning').

Basic organisation of cerebellar cortex

- The structural organisation of the cerebellum is uniform and similar to that of the cerebral hemispheres, having a thin layer of cortex, the deep white matter which contains the various cerebellar nuclei. Transversely orientated fissures divide the cerebellum into lobes.
- Two types of afferent fibres enter the cerebellar cortex:
  - climbing fibres originate in the contralateral inferior olivary nucleus and form powerful excitatory synapses with Purkinje cells
  - all other cerebellar afferents enter as mossy fibres and terminate in the granular layer.
- One type of efferent, Purkinje cell axons, leaves to convey information to the deep cerebellar nuclei.

Connections

- The superior peduncle connects the cerebellum to the midbrain and contains efferent fibres from the midbrain to the cerebellum and thalamus.

- The middle cerebral peduncle connects with the pons and contains axons of the pontine nuclei, relaying impulses from the higher centres to the cerebellum.
- The inferior cerebellar peduncle forms the connection between the medulla and cerebellum and carries fibres linking the vestibular nuclei, spinal cord and inferior olivary nuclei to the cerebellum.

Blood supply

- Via the posterior cerebral circulation from the vertebrobasilar system.
- The posterior inferior cerebellar arteries arise from the vertebral artery.
- The anterior inferior cerebellar arteries and the superior cerebellar arteries arise from the basilar artery.

Q80   Write short notes on the anatomy of the third cranial nerve nucleus

The third cranial nerve is also known as the oculomotor nerve. It has two motor nuclei: a main motor nucleus and an accessory parasympathetic nucleus called the Edinger–Westphal nucleus. The third nerve nucleus has no sensory output.

Main motor nucleus

- Situated in the midbrain at the level of the superior colliculus in the grey matter surrounding the cerebral aqueduct.
- Supplies levator palpebrae superioris muscle and all the extrinsic muscles of the eye except superior oblique and lateral rectus:
  - all these muscles are supplied by the ipsilateral nucleus except for superior rectus and levator palpebrae superioris. Superior rectus is supplied by the contralateral oculomotor nucleus and both levator palpebrae superioris muscles are supplied by a central group of cells, the central caudal nucleus.
- Outgoing nerve fibres pass anteriorly through the red nucleus to emerge on the anterior surface of the midbrain.
- Receives afferent corticonuclear fibres from both cerebral hemispheres and tectobulbar fibres from the superior colliculus, through which it receives information from the occipital cortex.
- The medial longitudinal fasciculus links the third cranial nerve nucleus to the nuclei of the fourth, sixth and eighth cranial nerves.

Accessory parasympathetic nucleus

- Lies immediately posterior to the main motor nucleus.
- Pre-ganglionic axons accompany other oculomotor axons to the orbit, where they synapse in the ciliary ganglion before supplying the sphincter pupillae and ciliary muscles.
- Receives corticonuclear fibres for the accommodation reflex and fibres from both pretectal nuclei for the direct and consensual light reflexes.

Q81 Write short notes on the third cranial nerve

Nuclei

- The third, or oculomotor nerve, is an entirely motor nerve and has no sensory nucleus.
- The main motor nucleus lies at the level of the superior colliculus in the periaqueductal grey matter of the midbrain.
- The accessory parasympathetic, or Edinger–Westphal, nucleus lies immediately posterior to this.

Course

- Outgoing motor fibres pass anteriorly through the red nucleus to emerge on the anterior surface of the midbrain, medial to the cerebral peduncle.
- The nerve passes between the posterior cerebral and superior cerebellar arteries before running forwards lateral to the posterior communicating artery within the subarachnoid space.
- The oculomotor nerve pierces the arachnoid and lies between the free and fixed edges of the tentorium cerebelli.
- On the lateral side of the posterior clinoid process the nerve perforates the dura to lie in the lateral wall of the cavernous sinus above the fourth cranial nerve:
  - the oculomotor nerve next runs forwards and receives a sensory branch from the ophthalmic division of the fifth cranial nerve and a sympathetic contribution from the internal carotid plexus
  - within the cavernous sinus the oculomotor nerve is crossed from its lateral side by the fourth cranial nerve. More distally it is crossed by the ophthalmic division of the fifth cranial nerve.
- The oculomotor nerve enters the orbit via the superior orbital fissure, within the tendinous ring, after dividing into superior and inferior divisions.

Superior division

- The superior division passes upwards lateral to the optic nerve to enter the superior rectus muscle at the junction of its proximal and middle thirds. The nerve passes through this muscle and terminates by supplying levator palpebrae superioris.

Inferior division

- The inferior division divides into three branches which supply the medial and inferior recti and the inferior oblique muscles:
  - the branch to medial rectus passes medially below the optic nerve to enter the lateral surface of the muscle at the junction between proximal and middle thirds
  - the branch to inferior oblique, which is the longest branch, passes forward close to the orbital floor and lateral to inferior rectus to enter the posterior border of inferior oblique
  - the branch to inferior rectus runs forward on the muscle's upper surface, entering it at the junction of its middle and proximal thirds.
- The nerve to inferior oblique gives rise to a short thick branch which passes to the ciliary ganglion, lateral to the optic nerve:
  - this branch contains parasympathetic fibres which synapse in the ciliary ganglion
  - post-ganglionic fibres to the sphincter pupillae and ciliary muscle fibres run in the short ciliary nerves.

Functions

- The third cranial nerve innervates the muscles that lift the upper eyelid and turn the globe upwards, downwards and medially together with those that constrict the pupil and cause accommodation.

Clinical notes

- Parasympathetic fibres run on the outside of the third cranial nerve and are vulnerable to compression by space-occupying lesions:
  - patients with pupil-involving oculomotor palsies should undergo neuroimaging
  - if painful, this is particularly urgent: posterior-communicating artery aneurysms classically present this way.

Q82   Write short notes on the fourth cranial nerve

Background

- The fourth cranial nerve, or trochlear nerve, is an entirely motor nerve which supplies the superior oblique muscle of the eye.
- It is the most slender of the cranial nerves and the only one to leave the brainstem dorsally.
- The primary action of the superior oblique on the globe is intorsion. Its secondary actions are depression, maximal in adduction, and abduction.

Nucleus

- The nucleus of the fourth cranial nerve lies in the anterior part of the periaqueductal grey matter in the midbrain. The nucleus lies at the level of the inferior colliculus and below the main motor nucleus of the third cranial nerve.
- The nucleus receives afferent corticonuclear fibres from both cerebral hemispheres and tectobulbar fibres from the superior colliculus, via which it is connected to the occipital cortex. The medial longitudinal fasciculus links the fourth nerve nucleus to the nuclei of the third, fourth and eighth cranial nerves.

Course

- After leaving the nucleus, efferent fibres pass posteriorly around the central grey matter to exit onto the posterior surface of the midbrain, where they immediately decussate.
- Lying in the subarachnoid space, the nerve passes laterally and forwards around the cerebral peduncle. It then pierces the arachnoid and perforates the dura just below the free border of the tentorium cerebelli, close to the posterior clinoid process.
- The nerve then passes forward in the lateral wall of the cavernous sinus, lying below the third cranial nerve and above the ophthalmic division of the fifth cranial nerve.

- At the anterior end of the cavernous sinus, the fourth cranial nerve crosses lateral to the third cranial nerve before entering the orbit via the superior orbital fissure, passing above the tendinous ring and medial to the frontal nerve.
- The fourth cranial nerve now passes medially above the origin of levator palpebrae superioris and enters the upper surface of superior oblique muscle as a series of small branches.

Clinical notes

- Fourth cranial palsy leads to vertical diplopia, which is often oblique.
- This diplopia is worse on downgaze, with gaze to the contralateral side and on ipsilateral head tilt.
- Patients with congenital fourth nerve palsies have increased vertical fusional ranges.

Q83   Give an account of the origin, course, relations and functions of the sixth cranial nerve

Overview

The sixth cranial nerve, or abducent nerve, is an entirely motor nerve which supplies the lateral rectus muscle of the eye and functions to abduct the globe.

Nucleus

- The nucleus of the sixth cranial nerve is situated beneath the facial colliculus in the floor of the upper part of the fourth ventricle, close to the midline.
- The nucleus receives afferent corticonuclear fibres from both cerebral hemispheres and tectobulbar fibres from the superior colliculus, via which it is connected to the occipital cortex.
- The medial longitudinal fasciculus links the sixth nerve nucleus to the nuclei of the third, fourth and eighth cranial nerves.

Course and relations

- The sixth cranial nerve has one of the longest intracranial courses of any cranial nerve.
- It emerges into the subarachnoid space from the anterior surface of the brainstem in a groove between the lower border of the pons and the medulla oblongata before running upwards, forwards and laterally to pierce the dura lateral to the dorsum sellae of the sphenoid bone.
- Near the apex of the petrous temporal bone, and on its upper border, the sixth cranial nerve makes an acute bend forward.
- Covered by endothelium, the sixth cranial nerve passes forward within the cavernous sinus, lying inferolateral to the internal carotid artery.
- The sixth cranial nerve enters the orbit through the superior orbital fissure, passing through the tendinous ring and lying between the two divisions of the third cranial nerve.

- The sixth cranial nerve ends by passing forwards to enter the medial surface of the lateral rectus muscle.

Clinical notes

Extranuclear palsy of the sixth cranial nerve results in esotropia and an ipsilateral abduction deficit.

Q84   Give an account of the structure and function of the primary visual cortex and its neuronal connections

Structure

- The primary visual cortex (PVC) or Brodman area 17 is situated either side of the calcarine sulcus on the medial aspect of the occipital lobe of both cerebral hemispheres. It extends from the parieto-occipital sulcus anteriorly to just posterolateral to the occipital pole.
- The middle and posterior cerebral arteries supply the PVC, the former anastomoses with the macular artery.
- Macroscopically the PVC is distinguished by the presence of a white stripe, the stria of Gennari, and microscopically this corresponds to layer IV, which is partly formed by terminating fibres of the optic radiation but mostly by intracortical connections.
- Like the cerebral cortex elsewhere, the PVC has a six-layered structure.
- Most cells are of a granular or stellate type with only a few pyramidal cells.

Connections

- Input to the PVC is principally from the ipsilateral lateral geniculate nucleus, whose cells synapse with stellate cells in layer IV:
    - the superior retina, and so the inferior visual field, projects to above the calcarine sulcus, the inferior retina to below
    - the macula projects posteriorly, the peripheral retina anteriorly
    - about 30% of the primary visual cortex represents the macula.
- The primary visual cortex is retinotopically mapped and corresponding retinal points from each eye project to adjacent columns, with each column receiving input from just one eye. These are called ocular dominance columns.
- Most cells in layer IV have 'centre–surround' type receptive fields.
- Cells from layer IV project to cells in adjacent layers which show increasingly complex receptive fields.
- Only cells after the first synapse in the visual cortex receive binocular input.
- Layers II and III of the primary visual cortex project to the secondary visual cortex (Brodman areas 18 and 19).

- Layer V projects to the superior colliculus.
- Layer VI contains predominantly pyramidal cells which project to the ipsilateral lateral geniculate nucleus.

Functions

- The PVC is concerned with conscious visual function.
- In conjunction with the secondary visual cortex and other cortical areas, it is involved in object recognition, colour vision, depth appreciation and movement detection.

Q85   Write short notes on the paranasal air sinuses

Overview

- All paranasal air sinuses are **present at birth** with the exception of the frontal sinus, which is rudimentary until age 2 and not fully formed until age 25.
- Considerable **variation** in size and shape between individuals.
- Lined by **pseudostratified columnar ciliated epithelium**.
- All lymphatic drainage is to submandibular nodes, except the sphenoidal and posterior ethmoidal sinuses, which drain into the retropharyngeal nodes.
- Important cause of **non-ocular eye pain**, for example in sinusitis, and a source from where **infective, inflammatory or neoplastic conditions can spread** to the orbit.
- In some individuals the sphenoid or ethmoidal sinuses may surround the **optic canal**. Sinusitis can consequently cause retrobulbar neuritis.
- Sinus surgery can potentially damage the optic nerve or contents of the orbit.

Frontal

- Lie within frontal bone.
- Innervated by supraorbital branch of the trigeminal nerve.
- Referred pain is to the skin of the scalp and forehead.
- Drain into the middle meatus of the nose via the frontonasal duct or ethmoidal infundibulum.

Ethmoidal

- Honeycomb of air cells within ethmoid bone but may extend into adjacent bones.
- Paper-thin **lamina papricea** separates from orbit.
- Ethmoidal sinusitis is commonest cause of **orbital cellulitis**.
- Innervated by anterior and posterior ethmoidal nerves and branches from the pterygopalatine ganglion.

- Drainage:
  - anterior group: middle meatus via ethmoidal infundibulum or fronto-nasal duct
  - middle group: middle meatus on or above bulla ethmoidalis
  - posterior group: superior meatus.

Maxillary

- Largest.
- Pyramid shaped in body of maxilla.
- Overlie the posterior five upper teeth and the roots of these often project into it. Orbital cellulitis can result from spread of dental abscesses by this route.
- **Blow-out fractures** involving the orbital floor may lead to prolapse of orbital fat into the maxillary sinus.
- Innervated by the anterior, middle and posterior superior alveolar and infraorbital nerves.
- Referred pain is to the upper teeth and skin of the cheek.
- Drain into the middle meatus through hiatus semilunaris.

Sphenoidal

- Within the body of the sphenoid bone but may extend into adjacent bones.
- Most variable between individuals.
- Referred pain is to the vertex of the scalp.
- Drain into the sphenoethmoidal recess.

Q86   Write short notes on the ventricles of the brain

Overview

- The cerebral ventricles are spaces within the brain that contain cerebrospinal fluid (CSF).
- Total adult CSF volume is 100–150 ml.
- CSF pressure is 8–10 cm H_2O.
- CSF is produced by the choroid plexus in all four ventricles and reabsorbed by the arachnoid granulations in the dural venous sinuses.
- The general shape of the ventricular system is shown in Figure 8.

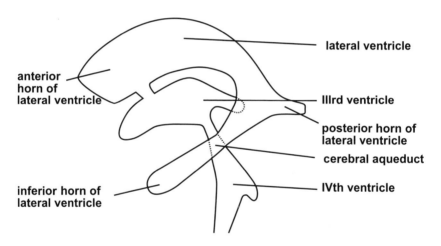

Figure 8   Lateral view of the cerebral ventricles.

Lateral ventricles

- The paired lateral ventricles are the largest of the ventricles.
- They lie within the cerebral hemispheres and each has a body: the thalamus and caudate nucleus form the floor, the corpus callosum the roof.
- The anterior horn projects forward in front of the intraventricular foramen of Monro: this connects the lateral ventricles to the third ventricle.
- The posterior horn projects into the occipital lobe, the inferior horn into the temporal lobe.

Third ventricle

- The third ventricle is a slit-shaped space in the midline between the two thalami and the hypothalamus.
- It is roofed by a double layer of pia mater, the tela choroidea, which contains choroid plexus.
- The cerebral aqueduct joins the third and fourth ventricles.

Fourth ventricle

- The tent-shaped fourth ventricle is inferior to the third ventricle.
- Its floor is formed by the pons and medulla and is diamond shaped; the superior and inferior medullary vela form the roof.
- The cerebellum lies posteriorly.
- Three openings in the roof of the fourth ventricle link it to the subarachnoid space:
  - the single midline foramen of Magendie to the cerebellomedullary cistern
  - the paired lateral foramen of Luschka to the pontine cistern.

Q87   Write short notes on the major photochemical events involved in phototransduction

Overview

- Phototransduction is the process by which light energy is converted into neuronal signals in the outer segments of photoreceptors.
- Rhodopsin, comprising the protein opsin linked by a Schiff linkage to the vitamin A derivative retinal, is the rod photopigment; iodopsin is the cone photopigment.
- Rhodopsin is in its resting state in the dark and photoreceptors are kept in a relatively depolarised state by the presence of cGMP [cyclic guanosine 3',5'-monophosphate] which holds open transmembrane sodium channels.
- In the light this situation reverses, causing a relative membrane hyper-polarisation.
- Phototransduction is similar in rods and cones: only rod phototransduction is discussed here.

Activation of rhodopsin

- Rhodopsin activation follows isomerisation of 11-*cis*-retinal to all-*trans*-retinal:
  - this is the only photoreaction in the cycle.
- During activation rhodopsin is converted to bathorhodopsin and then onto lumirhodopsin:
  - retinal isomerisation and photoreceptor bleaching is almost complete by the lumirhodopsin stage.
- Lumirhodopsin is then converted to metarhodopsin I and onto metarhodopsin II:
  - conversion of metarhodopsin I to II is the only reversible reaction in the series.
- The conformational change required for conversion of metarhodopsin I to II facilitates transducin binding (see below).
- Finally, metarhodopsin II is converted to metarhodopsin III, releasing all-*trans*-retinal following cleavage of the Schiff linkage.
- All-*trans*-retinal is reisomerised to 11-*cis*-retinal in the retinal pigment epithelium; the equivalent process for cones occurs in the neural retina.

Transducin

- Transducin is a G-protein with $\alpha\beta\gamma$ subunits.
- Transducin binds to the cytoplasmic loops of opsin after exposure of specific binding sites at the metarhodopsin II stage of rhodopsin activation.
- GDP [guanosine 5′-diphosphate] is bound to the transducin α subunit and during transduction it is replaced by GTP [guanosine 5′-triphosphate], which causes the transducin molecule to separate into α-GTP and $\beta\gamma$ subunits:
  - the $\beta\gamma$ subunits remain attached to the disc membrane
  - the α subunit combines with and activates phosphodiesterase (see below).
- Considerable amplification occurs at this stage: hundreds of transducin α-GTP are produced for every rhodopsin–photon interaction.

Phosphodiesterase

- Phosphodiesterase is an enzyme with $\alpha\beta2\gamma$ subunits.
- Phosphodiesterase is activated when its two γ subunits form a complex with two transducin α-GTP molecules.
- Activation leads to hydrolysis of cGMP to 5′-GMP and the resulting fall in cGMP causes closure of transmembrane sodium channels and membrane hyperpolarisation: this is the electrical response of photoreceptors to stimulation by light.

Q88　Write short notes on retinal neurotransmitters

The graded hyperpolarisation (analogue) photoreceptor response is transformed to a phasic (digital) ganglion response following processing within the neurosensory retina. There are several neurotransmitters involved in the transfer of information through synapses between the different retinal neural cell types.

Glutamatergic transmission

- **Glutamate** is tonically released by **photoreceptors and bipolar cells**.
- **Vesicular release** of glutamate occurs at **ribbon synapses**, specialised synapses used by cells using graded potentials. Synaptic release at ribbon synapses is higher compared to conventional synapses.
- Glutamate is loaded into synaptic vesicles by a vesicular glutamate transporter exploiting an electrochemical gradient created by a proton pump.
- **Exocytosis** is a **calcium-dependent** process.
- Glutamate acts on **ionotropic receptors** which gate cation channels at **sign-preserving synapses** (e.g. **photoreceptor-OFF bipolar cell synapse** uses the GluR5 or GluR6/7 receptors).
- **Sign-inversing synapses** rely on the **metabotropic**, G-protein coupled **mGluR6 receptor** which closes cation channels (e.g. **photoreceptor-ON bipolar cell synapse**).
- Glutamate is removed from the synapse by **excitatory amino acid transporters** present in most neural cell types and Muller glial cells in the neurosensory retina.

GABA [γ-aminobutyric acid] transmission

- GABA is synthesised from glutamate.
- Horizontal cells may use GABA for neurotransmission. 40% of amacrine cells are GABAergic. Interplexiform cells use GABA as their neurotransmitter.
- Release from amacrine cells is vesicular, from horizontal cells it may be vesicular or transporter-mediated.
- Binds to ionotropic (GABAA, GABAC) or metabotropic receptors (GABAB).
- Removed from synapse by transporter into glial cells.

Glycine transmission

- 40–50% of amacrine cells are glycinergic. The best characterised **glycinergic amacrine** cell is the **AII amacrine cell**.
- **AII cells** are narrow-field and form an **important part of the rod pathway**. Signals from rod bipolar cells are relayed to ON cone bipolar cells through gap junctions and through a chemical synapse to OFF cone bipolar cells.
- Glycine ionotropic receptors gate Cl channels and are classically thought to produce a hyperpolarising response.
- Glycine is removed from the synapse by the Glyt-1 glycine transporter into glycinergic amacrine cells.

Several other neurotransmitters have been identified in the retina (cholinergic-Starburst amacrine cells with a role in motion detection, dopamine, somato-statin, NO, substance P).

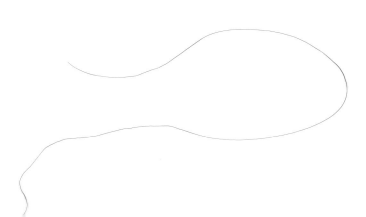

Q89 List the factors that determine corneal hydration

1 Stromal swelling pressure
2 Barrier function of the epithelium and endothelium
3 Endothelial pump
4 Evaporation from the corneal surface
5 Intraocular pressure.

Q90   Discuss the anatomical features of the extraocular muscles

There are six extraocular muscles in each eye: the four recti – medial, lateral, superior and inferior – and the two obliques – superior and inferior. These muscles originate from the bony orbit and insert into the globe which they move. Some consider levator palpebrae superioris to be an extraocular muscle but its function, elevation of the upper lid, is quite different to that of the muscles described below and it will not be discussed here.

The extraocular muscles are specialised striated muscles. Microscopically they have important differences from most striated muscles. Their epimysium (muscle sheath) is thinner, the fibres are less tightly packed (being separated by large amounts of connective tissue called perimysium) and the fibres are more rounded or oval in shape than in most striated muscles. Additionally, extra-ocular muscles are more vascular than any muscles except the myocardium.

The four recti muscles originate from the common tendinous ring, the annulus of Zinn, at the apex of the orbit and insert into the sclera anterior to the equator but posterior to the corneal limbus. The recti insert more or less at right angles to each other with each muscle occupying the position its name suggests – for example, the superior rectus is uppermost. The superior rectus is the longest muscle, then medial, then lateral, with inferior rectus being the shortest. The average length of the recti is 40 mm. The insertion of the medial rectus is closest (5.5 mm) to the corneoscleral limbus with inferior rectus inserting 6.5 mm, lateral rectus 6.9 mm and superior rectus 7.5 mm from the limbus. These insertions form the spiral of Tillaux. The oculomotor nerve supplies all the rectus muscles except lateral rectus, which is innervated by the abducent nerve.

Superior oblique originates superior medial to the optic canal. Its long tendon loops over the trochlear pulley in the anteromedial part of the roof of the orbit to insert into the posteromedial part of the sclera on the superior aspect of the globe, behind the equator and at an angle of $54°$ to the primary position. Inferior oblique originates from the floor of the orbit posterior to the orbital margin and lateral to the nasolacrimal canal. This muscle inserts into the sclera under the cover of the lateral rectus muscle on the posterolateral aspect of the globe at an angle of $55°$ to the primary position. The oculomotor nerve innervates inferior oblique, the trochlear nerve superior oblique.

Important relations of the extraocular muscles are as follows. Each oblique muscle passes below its corresponding rectus muscle. Levator palpebrae superioris runs above superior oblique and the two have fascial connections, facilitating coordinated movement. The optic nerve and ophthalmic artery enter the orbit within the tendinous ring. The ciliary ganglion lies between the optic nerve and lateral rectus. Part of the tendinous ring overlies the superior orbital fissure and (from superior to inferior) the superior division of the oculomotor nerve, the nasociliary nerve, the inferior division of the oculomotor nerve and the abducent nerve enter the orbit through this part. The lacrimal, frontal and trochlear nerves, together with the superior ophthalmic vein, pass above and the inferior ophthalmic vein passes below.

Q91   What are the Golgi apparatus? How are they involved in the secretion of proteins? Describe this process in relation to mast cells

Golgi apparatus are **intracellular organelles** found in all eukaryotic cells. Under the electron microscope they resemble a stack of plates and comprise layers of membrane-bound cisternae. Golgi apparatus often lie close to the cell nucleus. Many small vesicles surround the Golgi apparatus. Each Golgi stack has two distinct faces: a cis surface by which molecules enter and a trans surface through which they leave.

Functionally, the Golgi apparatus play an important role in **carbohydrate synthesis** and **post-translational protein modification**. They can be thought of as a sorting and dispatching station for products of the endoplasmic reticulum. Of particular note is their role in protein glycosylation. Transport vesicles carry molecules from one cisterna to the next within the Golgi apparatus.

Mast cells are specialised secretory cells. As such their Golgi apparatus are particularly well developed. In mast cells secretory vesicles containing histamine form by budding from areas of the Golgi apparatus which are clathrin-coated. The precise details of this process are poorly understood but it is thought that it involves the selective aggregation of secretory proteins. Mature vesicles result when the clathrin coat is removed from the newly formed vesicles.

Secretory vesicles then wait near the plasma membrane until their release, by endocytosis, is triggered. In mast cells release is triggered by immuno-globulin E (IgE) cross-linking on mast cells.

Q92 Compare and contrast the magnocellular and parvocellular pathways

The division of the human visual pathway into magnocellular and parvocellular pathways is based on neuroanatomical and neurophysiological studies.

It was in the striae of the lateral geniculate nucleus (LGN) that the neuroanatomical basis of this division was first described. Here layers 1 and 2 contain cells with large cell bodies, and are called the magnocellular layers, whereas layers 3 to 6 contain cells with small soma, called the parvocellular layers. Magnocellular and parvocellular layers of the LGN project to different sublayers of layer IV of the primary visual cortex: magnocellular layers to layer IVCα and parvocellular layers to IVCβ and IVA.

These anatomical differences reflect the different neurophysiological characteristics of the two pathways. Retinal efferents to the magnocellular pathway are mostly α type ganglions which have extensive dendritic trees, giving them large receptive fields. α ganglion cells exhibit non-linear spatial summation and respond in a transient or phasic manner. This pathway has a faster response than the parvocellular pathway and is most responsive to motion, flicker and light detection whereas the more slowly conducting parvocellular pathway conveys information on colour and fine detail as well as being integral for spatial discrimination. β ganglion cells are the major efferents to the parvocellular pathway and respond in a sustained manner and

Table 13 Differences between magnocellular and parvocellular ganglion cells

	Magnocellular pathway	*Parvocellular pathway*
Number	10% ganglion cells	80% ganglion cells
Cell body size	Large	Medium
Size of dendritic tree	Large	Small
Size of receptive field	Large	Small
Response	Transient	Sustained
Conduction speed	Rapid	Slower
Projection	Layers 1 and 2 of LGN and superior colliculus	Layers 3–6 of LGN only
Best stimulus	Large moving targets	Small targets
Origin	Concentrated around the fovea	Concentrated in fovea

exhibit linear spatial summation. They have smaller receptive fields and are slower to respond than α ganglion cells. Most rod photoreceptors synapse with α ganglion cells and most cone photoreceptors with β type ganglion cells. The magnocellular pathway therefore conveys most information from the retinal periphery whereas the parvocellular pathway conveys the majority of information from the foveal and parafoveal areas.

Approximately 80% of ganglion cells contribute to the parvocellular pathway and 10% to the magnocellular pathway.

Table 13 summarises the differences between magnocellular and parvocellular ganglion cells.

Q93   Write short notes on the development of the cornea

- Corneal development is thought to be induced by the lens and optic cup.
- Corneal development begins on day 33 after the lens cup has separated from the surface ectoderm. The layer of **surface ectoderm** that seals over the lens pit goes on to form the future corneal epithelium. Shortly after this a wave of mesenchyme passes over the optic cup margin and migrates centrally between the lens and future corneal epithelium to form the corneal endothelium. The future corneal endothelium is initially a bilayer.
- On around day 49 a second wave of mesenchyme begins migration from the optic cup margin and penetrates the space between the basal surface of the corneal epithelium and endothelium. These cells go on to form the fibroblasts that produce the corneal stroma.
- Both waves of mesenchyme are derived from the neural crest.
- By the third month the stroma has 25–30 layers, a thin Descemet's membrane is present and the endothelium has become a monolayer.
- Bowman's layer is the last of the five corneal layers to form.
- Corneal nerves are present by five months.
- The cornea has reached its adult form by seven months.
- The cornea is not transparent throughout development but becomes so gradually as its structure becomes more ordered.
- Final corneal diameter is reached by about 2 years of age. The optic cup diameter determines the final corneal diameter.

Q94   Write short notes on the prenatal development of the lens. Use annotated diagrams where possible

- The lens forms from **surface ectoderm** covering the head of the embryo. Patches of cells that lie on either side of the head express the transcription factor *Pax-6* and have a 'lens-forming bias'.
- The optic vesicles appear as outpouchings from the diencephalon (day 25) and grow into close apposition to the surface ectoderm. They induce the ectodermal cuboidal cells to elongate and become columnar, forming the **lens placode** (day 27).
- The **lens pit** appears in the lens placode and deepens by a process of differential cellular elongation and multiplication (day 29). This causes the lens placode and the adjacent cells of the optic vesicle to buckle inward, transforming the latter into a two-layered optic cup.
- As the lens pit continues to invaginate, the stalk of cells that connect the lens to the surface ectoderm undergoes apoptosis. The resulting sphere consists of a single layer of cuboidal cells within a basement membrane, known as the **lens vesicle** (day 33). The apices of the cells are towards the lumen of the vesicle, with their bases at the periphery.
- The defect over the lens vesicle heals without scarring by adjacent *Pax-6* expressing cells which become the corneal and conjunctival epithelial cells.
- The posterior cells of the lens vesicle elongate and obliterate the lumen of the lens vesicle to form the **primary lens fibres**. They make up the embryonic nucleus which occupies the central area of the adult lens.
- The monolayer of cuboidal cells anteriorly is referred to as the **lens epithelium**.
- The basement membrane becomes the **lens capsule**.
- At about 7 weeks of gestation, cells of the lens epithelium near the lens's equator begin to multiply rapidly and elongate into **secondary lens fibres**. The anterior aspect of each lens fibre grows anteriorly under the lens epithelium, whereas the posterior aspect grows towards the posterior pole immediately under the posterior capsule. The lens fibres meet anteriorly and posteriorly to form the anterior and posterior sutures, which are Y-shaped in the embryonic lens.
- Initially the fetal lens's anterior–posterior diameter exceeds its equatorial diameter. As more secondary fibres are added, this situation reverses.
- The hyaloid artery gives rise to a series of small capillaries that anastomose with choroidal and long ciliary arteries to form a vascular

capsule, the **tunica vasculosa lentis**, providing the rich nutrient supply necessary for the rapid growth of the lens during development. This capsule regresses shortly before birth.

- The lens at birth is avascular and insensate.

Q95 Write short notes on the early development of the vitreous

- Between weeks 4 and 5 the lentoretinal space becomes filled with fibrils, mesenchymal cells and vascular channels. These elements constitute the **primary vitreous**. The mesenchymal cells and vascular channels derive from the hyaloid artery, which enters the optic cup through the choroidal fissure. The hyaloid artery gives rise to a series of small capillaries that anastomose with choroidal and long ciliary arteries to form a vascular capsule, the **tunica vasculosa lentis**, providing the rich nutrient supply necessary for the rapid growth of the lens during development.
- From 6 to 12 weeks the avascular **secondary vitreous** is deposited behind the primary vitreous, which slowly regresses leaving Cloquet's canal as its remnant, whereas the tunica vasculosa lentis regresses shortly before birth.
- The **tertiary vitreous** forms by condensation of the primary vitreous.

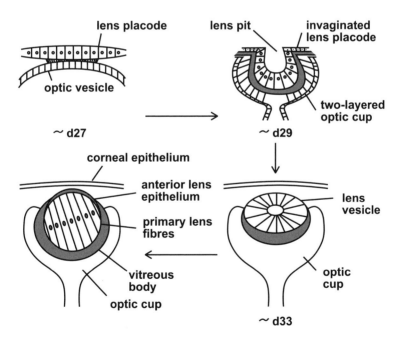

Figure 9 Development of the lens and vitreous.

Q96   Write short notes on the development of the retina

- The **optic vesicle** is fully formed by day 25 of gestation and after it invaginates the thickened inner invaginated layer, known as the retinal disc, is destined to differentiate into the neural retina whereas the outermost layer of the optic cup is destined to become the retinal pigment epithelium (RPE). There is a sharp transition between these two layers at the optic cup margin.
- The outer layer, or future RPE, consists of pseudostratified columnar cells. Pigment granules are present from as early as the third week of gestation. These cells continue to divide late into fetal life. The basal lamina of the RPE is incorporated into Bruch's membrane.
- The primitive neural retina is formed from the inner layer of the optic cup and consists of an outer nuclear zone and an inner marginal (or acellular) zone. The outer nuclear zone is homogeneous to the proliferative neuroepithelium of the neural tube.
- Mitotic activity in the primitive neural retina is greatest in the outer part of the outer nuclear zone and is completed by 15 weeks. Differentiation begins as mitosis ends. Differentiation is initiated in the marginal zone, commencing at the posterior pole and progressing in a centrifugal manner.
- From about 7 weeks' gestation newly formed cells migrate vitread from the nuclear zone into the marginal zone to form the inner neuroblastic layer. From this time the nuclear zone becomes known as the outer neuroblastic layer.
- The inner neuroblastic layer goes on to produce ganglion and amacrine cells whereas the outer neuroblastic layer gives rise to horizontal and bipolar elements.
- Photoreceptors are thought to be derived from cilia found in the outer nuclear zone.

Lamination is essentially complete by four and a half months and the ora serrata formed by six months.

Index

Page numbers in *italics* refer to tables or illustrations.

α-agonists, and intraocular pressure (IOP) 9
α-blockers, and blood pressure 17
abductant (sixth cranial) nerve 122–3
acarbose 16
accommodation 113
accommodation reflex, and convergence
    movements 104
aqueous–vitreous barrier 4
active secretion 101
acuity, classification 95
adaptation 85–6
    dark adaptation 83–4, 85–6
    light adaptation 85
age, and drug metabolism 6
AIDS (acquired immunodeficiency
    syndrome) 35–6
air-puff tonometers 100
allograft rejection 67
aminoglycosides, side-effects 18
amniocentesis 57
angina 61
angiotensin II antagonists, and blood pressure
    17
angiotensin-converting enzyme (ACE)
    inhibitors 17
ankylosing spondylitis 66
antibiotics
    bacterial resistance 48
    metabolism 5–6
    mode of action 45, 47
    side-effects 18
antigen recognition 65–6
    role of T-lymphocytes 68
antihypertensive agents 17
apoptosis 45
    and neoplasm formation 55–6
applanation tonometry 100
aqueous drainage 25
    anterior chamber structures 110–11
aqueous secretion 101
    drug actions 101–2
    mechanism for active control 101
    mechanisms for passive control 101–2

Arden ratio 88
arteritis 37, 61
ascorbic acid 82
atherosclerosis 60
    pathogenesis 40–1, 72
autoclaving techniques 52
autonomic nervous system, sympathetic v.
    parasympathetic 29

β-agonists, and intraocular pressure (IOP) 9
β-blockers 17
    and intraocular pressure (IOP) 9
    side-effects 14
bacteria 53
    antibiotic resistance 48
    gram-positive/negative classification 47
    tissue destruction mechanisms 34
Behçets disease 66
biguanides 15
birdshot choroidoretinopathy 66
Bjerrum screen 98
blind spots 98
blood supply
    cerebellum 116
    conjunctiva 77
    cortex 78
    eyelids 76–7
    and flow autoregulation 28
    iris and ciliary body 76
    lens and cornea 76
    visual pathway 78
blood–aqueous barrier 4
blood–retinal barrier 4
blow-out fractures 127
Bowman's layer 140
Brodman area 17 *see* primary visual cortex

calcium channel blockers, and blood pressure 17
canal of Schlemm 110, *110*
carbohydrate synthesis 137
carbonic anhydrase inhibitors 12, 32
    and intraocular pressure (IOP) 9
    systemic agents 12
    topical agents 13

carcinomas *see* neoplasms
cataracts
  diabetes-related 81
  and UV light exposure 92
cell activities
  apoptosis 45
  carbohydrate synthesis 137
  glucose metabolism 73, 81
  immune response 62
  oxidative phosphorylation 73, 81
  protein glycolisation 137
  water transfer 31–2
cellulitis 126–7
cerebellum 115–16
  blood supply 116
  connections 115–16
cerebral ventricles 128–9
cerebrospinal fluid (CSF) 128–9
chlamydia *53*
chorionic villus sampling (CVS) 57
chromosomal translocation 59
ciliary bodies 112–13
  anatomy 112–13, *112*
  aqueous drainage 111
  blood supply 76
  functions 113
circulatory system
  autoregulation 28
  diabetes and vascular changes 39
  and hypertension 72
  occlusive diseases 60–1
  see also blood supply
colour constancy 106
colour perception 96, 105–6
complement cascade 62
  and immunoglobulin function 63, *64*
confidence interval (CI) 1
conjugation 5, 48
conjunctiva
  blood supply 77
  function 109
  innervation 109
  structure 109
  UV light exposure 92
contact lenses
  drug-impregnated 3
  and infection control 50–1
  Pseudomonas aeruginosa infections 49
contrast detection 96
Coppock cataract 54
cornea
  aqueous drainage 110–11

  blood supply 76
  development 140
  hydration 134
  protective functions 3–4
  ulceration 42–3
  UV light exposure 92
corneal wedge 110
cortical control
  eye movements 96, 103
  visual perception 96–7
corticosteroids, side-effects 19, *20*
cranial nerves
  oculomotor (third) nerve 117–19
  trochlear (fourth) nerve 120–1
  abductant (sixth) nerve 122–3
crystallins 80
cycloplegic agents 11, *11*
cytochrome P450 5
cytolysis 62

dark adaptation 83–4, 85–6
descemetocele 42–3
Descemet's membrane 110, 140
diabetes
  cataract formation 81
  drug actions 15–16
  vascular changes 39
diplopia 121
diuretics, mode of action 31–2
DNA (deoxyribonucleic acid)
  amplification techniques 58
  and bacterial resistance 48
  and viral replication 46
Down syndrome, ocular features 59
drug actions, on pupil dilation 7–8
drug administration methods
  bolus v. continuous 4
  drug-impregnated contact lenses 3
  injections 3
drug interactions 6
drug metabolism 5–6
drug penetration, determining factors 3–4

echography 57
Edinger–Westphal (accessory parasympathetic)
  nucleus 117, 118
electro-oculograms (EOGs) 88
electroretinograms (ERGs) 88–9
  pERG (pattern ERG) 89
embolisms 60
endocytosis 33

endothelial pump   134
endotoxins   34
enzyme systems, and free radical damage   44
esotropia   123
ethmoidal sinuses   126–7
exotoxins   34
extraocular muscles
   actions   79
   anatomical features   135–6
eye movements   79, 135–6
   cortical control   96
   supranuclear control   103–4
eyelids
   blood supply   76–7
   structure   107–8, 107

fetal development see prenatal development
fetoscopy   57
fluoroquinolone   49
free radical damage
   retinal photoreceptors   44, 92
   and UV light exposure   92
frontal sinuses   126
fusion inhibitors   22

GABA (γ-aminobutyric acid) transmission
   132
galactosaemia   81
ganglion cells
   anatomical classification   26
   connections   26–7
   physiological classification   26
   visual pathways   138–9, 138
Ganz field screen   98
gene abnormalities
   and bacterial resistance   48
   detection mechanisms   58
   and drug metabolism   6
   mechanisms   59
   and neoplasms   55
genetic linkage   54
giant cell arteritis (GCA)   37, 61
glaucoma, and visual field   98
gliclazide   15
glucocorticoid receptors   30
glucose metabolism   73
   in the lens   81
glutamatergic transmission   132
glutathione concentration levels   82
glycine transmission   133
glycolysis   73, 81
Goldmann applanation tonometer   100

Goldmann perimeter   99
Golgi apparatus   137
gram staining   47

HAART (highly active antiretroviral
   therapy)   22
histocompatibility antigens   65–6
   disease associations   66
HIV (human immunodeficiency virus), treatment
   strategies   21–2
HLA (human leukocyte antigens)   65–6
Humphrey perimeter   99
hydrostatic pressure   31
hyperacuity   95
hypersensitivity response   34
hypertension
   drug treatments   17
   histology   72

immune response
   and allograft rejection   67
   complement cascade   62
   histocompatibility antigens   65–6
   immunoglobulin functions   63, 64, 109
   innate v. adaptive mechanisms   70–1
   role of conjunctiva   109
immunoglobulins   63, 64, 109
indentation tonometry   100
infection control
   MRSA precautions   50–1
   sterilisation principles   52
infrared light exposure   91–2
innervation, pupil   7
intranuclear opthalmoplegia (INO)   104
intraocular pressure (IOP)   9, 25
   drug actions   9–10
   measurement   100
investigations, electrophysiological
   techniques   88–90
iodopsin   130
ionising radiation, pathological effects   38
iris
   blood supply   76
   innervation   118–19
iris processes   111

keratitis
   following contact lens use   49
   following infections   42
   following radiotherapy   38
kinetic testing   99

lacrimal glands   114
lateral geniculate nucleus (LGN)   27
  blood supply   78
  magnocellular v. parvocellular pathways
     138–9, *138*
  neuroanatomy   94
lens
  blood supply   76
  carbohydrate metabolism   81
  crystallins   80
  oxidation protective mechanisms   82
  prenatal development   141–2
  UV light exposure   92
LGN *see* lateral geniculate nucleus
Li–Fraumeni syndrome   55
light adaptation   85
lignocaine, metabolism   6
lipid auto-oxidation   44
lobulated tubuloacinarstructure   114
lymphatic drainage   126–7

macular degeneration, and UV light exposure
  92
magnocellular visual pathways   138–9, *138*
MALT (mucosa-associated lymphoid tissue)
  109
maxillary sinuses   127
Meibomian glands   108
metformin   15
miotics   8
mitochondria   73
MLF (medial longitudinal fasciculus)
  lesions   104
  vertical gaze control   103
motion detection   96
MRSA (methicillin-resistant *Staphylococcus aureus*),
  precautions   50–1
Muller's muscle *107*, 108
multiple sclerosis   104
muscarinic agonists, and intraocular pressure
  (IOP)   9
muscle groups, extraocular muscles   79
mydriatics   8

Na–K ATPase inhibitors, and intraocular pressure
  (IOP)   10
neonatal development
  cornea   140
  and drug metabolism   6
  lens   142
neoplasms   69
  AIDS-related   36

genetic mechanisms   55–6
  local effects   69
  systemic effects   69
neurophysiology
  fourth cranial nerve   120–1
  ganglion cells   26–7
  magnocellular v. parvocellular visual
    pathways   138–9, *138*
  pupil   7
  sixth cranial nerve   122–3
  third cranial nerve   117–19
  visual pathway   93–4
neurotransmitters, retina   132–3
nitrates, and blood pressure   17
nystagmus   104

object identification   96–7
occlusive disease   60–1
ocular barriers   3–4
oculomotor (third cranial) nerve   117–19
  clinical presentations   119
  motor nuclei   117
oedema, in heart failure   31
oncogene activation   55–6
opponent theory   105–6
opportunistic infections, AIDS-related   35
opsonisation   62
optic chiasma
  blood supply   78
  neuroanatomy   93
optic nerve
  blood supply   78
  neuroanatomy   93
optic neuritis, and visual field   98
optic radiation
  blood supply   78
  neuroanatomy   94
optic tract
  blood supply   78
  neuroanatomy   93–4
orbit, bony anatomy   74–5
orbital cellulitis   126–7
osmotic agents, and intraocular pressure (IOP)
  9, 101
osmotic pressure   31–2
ouabain   32
oxidative phosphorylation   44, 73

paracetamol, metabolism   5–6
paranasal air sinuses   126–7
parapontine reticular formation (PPRF)   103

parasympathetic nervous system 29
parvocellular visual pathways 138–9, 138
pattern (ERGs) 89
Perkins tonometer   100
phagocytosis 33
phosphodiesterase   131
photo-oxidation   44
photoreceptors 23–4
   adaptation mechanisms   83–4, 85–6
   endocytosis   33
   free radical damage   44
   oxygen requirements *in vitro*   44
   phototransduction   130–1
   retinal transmitters   131–3
phototransduction   130–1
pingueculae, and UV light exposure   92
pinocytosis   33
polymerase chain reactions (PCR)   58
polymyalgia rheumatica   61
positive predictive value (PPV)   2
pregnancy, prenatal testing   57
prenatal development
   cornea   140
   lens   141–2
   retina   144
   vitreous   143
prenatal testing   57
pressure ulcers *see* ulcers
prevalence, screening measures   2
primary visual cortex   124–5
   connections   124–5
   functions   125
   neuroanatomy   94, 124
primary visual cortex (V_1)   96–7
protease inhibitors   21
protein glycolisation   137
proteinuria   39
Pseudomonas aeruginosa   49
pterygia, and UV light exposure   92
pupillary responses
   innervation   7, 7
   pharmacological modification   7–8
pursuit movements   96, 103

radiotherapy, pathological effects   38
repaglinide   15
retina
   blood supply   78
   neuroanatomy   93
   neurotransmitters   132–3
   UV light exposure   92
   vascular occlusion   61

retinal pigment epithelium (RPE)   87
retinoblastomas, genetic mechanism   55
retinotopic organisation, visual pathway   93–4
reverse transcriptase inhibitors (RTIs)   21
rhodopsin   130
ribbon synapses   132
RNA (ribonucleic acid), and viral replication   46
Robertsonian translocation   59
rods and cones
   adaptation mechanisms   83–4, 85–6
   biochemical aspects compared 24
   and endocytosis   33
   free radical damage   44
   functional/organisational aspects compared 24
   phototransduction   130–1
   retinal neurotransmission   132–3
   structural features compared 23

saccadic eye movements   96, 103
Schiotz tonometer   100
Schwalbe's line   110
scleral spur   111
scotomas   98
screening tests
   positive predictive value (PPV)   2
   sensitivity measures   2
   specificity measures   2
secretagogues   15
sensitivity measures   2
sinuses   126–7
sinusitis   126
skeletal muscle v. extraocular muscle   79
sorbitol pathway   81
specificity measures   2
sphenoidal sinuses   127
standard deviation (SD)   1
standard error of the mean (SEM)   1
staphylomas   43
static testing   99
statistical measures   1
stereoacuity   95
sterilisation   52
steroid receptors   30
strokes
   causes   60–1
   lesions   104
   pathogenesis   40–1, 61
supranuclear control systems   103–4
   pursuit movements   96, 103
   saccadic movements   96, 103
   vergence movements   104
   vestibular movements   104

sympathetic nervous system *29*
sympathetic ophthalmia   66
systemic anti-hypertensive agents, and intraocular
    pressure (IOP)   10

T-lymphocytes   68
tear production   109, 114
thrombosis   60
tonometry   100
trabecular meshwork   110, *110*
transducin   131
transduction   48
transferrin   82
transformation   48
translocation   59
transplants, allograft rejection   67
trichromatic theory   105–6
trochlear (fourth cranial) nerve   120–1
    clinical presentations   121
tumour suppressor genes   56
tunica vasculosa lentis   142

ulcers
    causes   42
    pathogenesis   42–3
ultrafiltration   101–2

UV light exposure   44, 91–2
    and neoplasms   55
uveoscleral drainage   25

vasculitides   60–1
vasospasms   61
ventricles   128–9
VEPs (visually evoked potentials)   89–90
vergence movements   104
Vernier acuity   95
vertical diplopia   121
vestibular movements   104
viruses *53*
    replication   46
visual acuity   98
    classification   95
visual cortex, blood supply   78
visual field   98
    measurement techniques   98–9
visual pathway
    blood supply   78
    magnocellular v. parvocellular   138–9, *138*
    retinotopic organisation   93–4

water transfer through tissues   31–2
Wegener's disease   60